CLIENT-CENTERED
OCCUPATIONAL THERAPY

CLIENT-CENTERED
OCCUPATIONAL THERAPY

Edited by Mary Law, PhD, OT(C)

McMaster University
Hamilton, Ontario
Canada

SLACK Incorporated, 6900 Grove Road, Thorofare, NJ, 08086

Publisher: John H. Bond
Editorial Director: Amy E. Drummond
Creative Director: Linda Baker
Assistant Editor: Elisabeth DeBoer

Client-Centered Occupational Therapy/edited by Mary Law
  p. cm
  Includes bibliographical references and index.
  ISBN 1-55642-264-4 (alk. paper)
  1. Occupational therapy. 2. Therapist and patient. I. Law, Mary C.
  [DNLM: 1. Occupational Therapy--methods. 2. Nondirective Therapy.
 WB 555 C636 1998]
 RM735.C59 1998
 615.8'515--dc21
 DNLM/DLC
 for Library of Congress   98-17783
                       CIP

Printed in the United States of America
Published by: SLACK Incorporated
      6900 Grove Road
      Thorofare, NJ 08086-9447 USA
      Telephone: 609-848-1000 or 856-848-1000
      Fax: 609-853-5991 or 856-853-5991
      http://www.slackinc.com

Contact SLACK Incorporated for more information about other books in this field or about the availability of our books from distributors outside the United States.

Last digit is print number: 10 9 8 7 6 5 4 3 2

NOTE TO THE READER

Although we have chosen to use the American spelling of the word centered in the title of this book, the Canadian or British spelling has been retained throughout the text to reflect the origin of the concept of Client-Centred Occupational Therapy.

DEDICATION

To Brian, Michael, Geoffrey, and Andrew.

CONTENTS

ACKNOWLEDGMENTS

I want to thank all the contributors to this book. Their experiences, wisdom and ideas are reflected in each chapter. I am fortunate to work with many colleagues and friends who provide support and lively discussion everyday. Thanks in particular to everyone in the Neurodevelopmental Clinical Research Unit and in the School of Rehabilitation Science at McMaster University. A very special thank you to the people at SLACK Incorporated—Peter Slack, John Bond, Amy Drummond, Debra Christy, and all who have had a part in putting this book together. From the time that Amy first talked to me about the book until today, they have always provided excellent guidance and support. And always—to Brian, Michael, Geoffrey and Andrew—your love and support make everything worthwhile.

CONTRIBUTORS

Sue Baptiste, MHSc, OT(C), is Associate Professor in the School of Rehabilitation Science at McMaster University, Hamilton, Canada. She is one of the authors of the Canadian Occupational Performance Measure (COPM), a client-centred assessment for occupational therapists. Her research and educational interests center on problem-based and self-directed learning and the use of self-assessment by occupational therapists to improve their practice.

Carolyn Baum, PhD, OTR/C, FAOTA, is the Elias Michael Director and Assistant Professor of Occupational Therapy and Neurology at Washington University School of Medicine, St. Louis, MO. She has served as President of the American Occupational Therapy Association, President of the National Board for Certification of Occupational Therapy, and on committees at the National Center for Medical Rehabilitation Research at the National Institutes of Health and at the Institute of Medicine. Her research interests centre on the impact of cognitive impairment on occupational performance in daily life.

Jo Clark, BSc, OT(C) is Clinical Coordinator, Occupational Therapy Services, Vancouver Hospital, UBC Site and Clinical Associate Professor, School of Rehabilitation Sciences, University of British Columbia, Vancouver, Canada. She also has a private practice centred on stress disability and return to work.

Virginia G. Fearing, BSc, OT(C) is Professional Practice Leader, Occupational Therapy at Vancouver Hospital & Health Sciences Centre in Vancouver, British Columbia. She is also Clinical Professor in the Occupational Therapy Division of the School of Rehabilitation Sciences at the University of British Columbia.

Karen Whalley Hammell, MSc, OT(C) is currently completing an interdisciplinary doctorate (Rehabilitation Sciences, Anthropology, Sociology) at the University of British Columbia.

Mary Law, PhD, OT(C) is Professor in the School of Rehabilitation Science and Director of the Neurodevelopmental Clinical Research Unit at McMaster University, Hamilton, Canada. She is also one of the authors of the Canadian Occupational Performance Measure (COPM). Her research interests centre on environmental factors which support daily life participation of children with disabilities, measurement of occupational performance, and transfer of research information into practice.

Leonard N. Matheson, PhD is a psychologist who believes that occupational therapists have tremendous potential to extend the effect of rehabilitation through their global perspective on the person. His research interests range from the development of functional assessment techniques to exploration of the subtle first principles and central organizing characteristics of therapeutic change. He teaches and performs research in the Occupational Therapy Program at Washington University in St. Louis.

Mary Ann McColl, PhD, OT(C) is Professor of Rehabilitation Therapy and Community Health and Epidemiology at Queen's University, Kingston, Canada. She is one of the authors of the Canadian Occupational Performance Measure (COPM), as well as an author of several books on occupational therapy and disability.

Jennifer Mills, BHSc, OT(C) is an occupational therapist, self-employed in a community-based practice.

Nancy Pollock, MSC, OT(C) is Associate Professor in the School of Rehabilitation Science and Co-investigator, Neurodevelopmental Clinical Research Unit at McMaster University, Hamilton, Canada. She is one of the authors of the Canadian Occupational Performance Measure (COPM). Her practice and research are with children with special needs.

Sarah Rochon, MSc(T), OT(C) is Assistant Clinical Professor in the School of Rehabilitation Science at McMaster University. Her career as an occupational therapist has spanned over two decades, and has included roles as an educator, consultant, clinician and manager. Her interests include clinical reasoning, adult mental health, and professional and organizational development.

Sue Stanton, MA, OT(C) is Senior Instructor in the Occupational Therapy Program at the University of British Columbia, with special interests in stroke rehabilitation, organizational change, and the application of occupational therapy theory to practice.

Elizabeth (Liz) Townsend, PhD, OT(C) has participated since 1980 in developing all Canadian guidelines for client-centred occupational therapy practice, and was Editor of the latest guidelines, *Enabling Occupation: An Occupational Therapy Perspective*, published in 1997 by the Canadian Association of Occupational Therapists. She is currently a founding member, Associate Professor and Director of the School of Occupational Therapy, and Coordinator of Studies on Occupation, Faculty of Health Professions, Dalhousie University in Halifax, Nova Scotia, Canada.

PREFACE

Occupational therapy, at its best, is client-centred. The person receiving occupational therapy services leads the way in making decisions about the focus and the nature of therapy intervention. The relationship between that person, his or her family, and the occupational therapist is a collaborative partnership whose goal is to enhance occupational performance, health and well-being. Client-centred occupational therapy promotes participation, exchange of information, client decision-making, and respect for choice. Through a client-centred occupational therapy service, satisfaction and functional outcomes improve. Time and resources are maximized because therapy focuses on the issues which are most important to the person and his or her family.

If a client-centred approach to occupational therapy can achieve all these goals, why don't all therapists practice from that perspective? There's a very obvious reason—to be client-centred is challenging. This model of service delivery is challenging because of time and resource pressures, because of the structure of our health care system, and because every client and his or her family is unique. Another challenge is not being certain of what to do—what are the skills that I need, how should I do assessment, what does client-centred occupational therapy look like?

My hope in writing this book is to provide information and ideas to assist occupational therapists in meeting the challenge of practising in a client-centred manner. I have purposefully combined theoretical and practical information within the same volume (and often the same chapter) to encourage the implementation of theory (ideas) into practice. The book begins with an historical perspective on client-centred practice from its origins with Carl Rogers. In Chapters 1 and 2, important concepts of client-centred practice are discussed, and evidence is provided to illustrate the positive impact of this service delivery method on client satisfaction and functional outcome. Chapter 3 provides information about how a client-centred practice fits with the health care system today. In Chapter 4, a case study of the evolution of client-centred occupational therapy in Canada is presented. This case study illustrates the results of a nationally-based focus on the development of client-centred guidelines for occupational therapy practice. Chapters 5 through 8 demonstrate the application of client-centred concepts throughout the occupational therapy process, including assessment and intervention. Specific examples are included to provide guidance to therapists for implementation into practice. Finally, Chapter 9 provides information and reflective exercises to enable occupational therapists to contemplate issues of ethics and client-centred practice.

This is the first book that I have edited, so everything is new to me. It's exciting, yet formidable. The process of writing and editing took much longer than expected, but the book is better because of that time for reflection and growth. I look forward to hearing from you as you read and use this book. I welcome your comments.

Mary Law
April 20, 1998
Cambridge, Ontario, Canada

chapter

CLIENT-CENTRED OCCUPATIONAL THERAPY

MARY LAW, PHD, OT(C), JENNIFER MILLS, BHSC, OT(C)

"During my two hour visit with my 92 year old, fully-aware grandfather, I experience what is not a grand revelation to many: hospitals are sorely impersonal." L. M. Cherniak, Toronto Globe & Mail, July 6, 1994

"They tried to teach him how to butter his toast. I can assure you, he has never buttered his toast in his entire life. What a waste; every day was a new day, every day was a new experience. A lot of time and attention was spent on things like teaching him how to dress himself. It would take him two hours to dress on his own, but with my assistance, he could do it in ten minutes." Swanson (1997), p. 51

As we approach the end of the 20th century, health care in North America and around the world is changing rapidly. Rising costs, changing definitions of health, a need to move services from institutions to communities, increased interest by consumers in directing their health care, and increased prevalence of chronic disability have led to significant changes in how health care is defined and delivered. All of these changes have had an impact on the practice of occupational therapy. The focus of occupational therapy practice is broadening, with less practice in institutions and increasing work in communities. Occupational therapists, like all health service providers, are searching methods of providing service that truly meet the needs of people seeking occupational therapy intervention.

The United States spends 15% of its gross national product on the provision of health care. Rising costs, along with dissatisfaction in health outcomes, have led to a revolution in the way that health care is managed and provided. Managed care systems, in which all health services for a set population are managed and contracted, have come to dominate the health care system in many parts of the United States. While it has been stated that the goal of managed care is quality outcomes at a manageable cost, there have been many criticisms that services, including rehabilitation and occupational therapy services, have been severely restricted in order to contain costs. In Canada, although health care spending is significantly less, at 8% of the gross national product, there have also been increasing restraint and significant changes in the health care system. Many provinces in Canada have restructured the health system and appointed regional health boards with a fixed budget to manage health care for that community. Hospital beds have been decreased, and hospital budgets have been cut. In some instances, these costs have been put into community care, but this has not always been the case.

The definition of health from the World Health Organization and the Ottawa Charter states that health is more than the absence of disease and that health includes life satisfaction and a sense of well-being (Epp, 1986). The Ottawa Charter for Health Promotion, supported by 38 countries, discusses health as a positive concept and stresses the need for health promotion, the creation of supportive and ecological environments, community action programs, and health services that promote health and well-being. Health has become a concept that we believe is created by people and involves active participation in daily activities. Concomitant with changing definitions of health is a recognition that the prevalence of chronic disability has increased dramatically over the past several decades. People with disabilities are living longer, are aging, and are living in the community. Their ability to participate in day-to-day community activities is an increasing concern.

People receiving occupational therapy and other rehabilitation services are quite rightly demanding to be partners in service provision. Consumer movements have increased our awareness that we, as citizens, have a right to participate in the way that care is provided. Increasingly, people seeking occupational therapy services want to be responsible for the services that are provided and to have autonomy in making decisions about these services (Haiman, 1995). Occupational therapists support the active engagement of people in their chosen occupations of daily life. It would seem natural, therefore, that consumers should be directing occupational therapy service.

There is evidence, however, that clients of occupational therapy are not leading the way in decision making about therapy intervention. Neistadt (1995) conducted a survey of 269 occupational therapy directors in adult physical rehabilitation facilities to determine the methods by which the goals of occupational therapy were developed. The findings of this study indicate that the vast majority of respondents used primarily informal interviews to identify client priorities. This method may not lead to the development of specific occupational goals. Neistadt found that the goals that were set were vague and did not cite specific occupations that were meaningful for that client. In another study, Northen, Rust, Nelson, and Watts (1995) audiotaped the initial evaluation sessions of 30 occupational therapists in adult physical rehabilitation practice settings. Using set criteria to evaluate the participation of clients in goal setting, Northen et al. found that percentages of these criteria that were used ranged from 17.4% to 78.9% with an average of 43.3%. Criteria that were rarely met included discussing with the individual how they will participate in goal setting, introducing how to explore concerns, asking people to establish the priority of their concerns, explaining the cooperative role of the client in goal identification, incorporating the client-stated concerns in the exploration of therapy goals, and documenting clients rating of the significance of their goals.

These experiences in occupational therapy are similar to experiences in other health care professions. For example, Johnson (1993) conducted interviews with four people with disabilities who live in the community to discuss their experiences with physiotherapy services. The results of this study indicate that the people receiving these services perceived physiotherapists as insensitive, condescending, and more focused on solving problems than tailoring therapy intervention to meet the needs of the person living independently in the community. Moorehead and Winefield (1991) found that empathetic responding to patients did not increase after intensive counseling training for medical students. Students invariably focused on solving medical problems instead of focusing on the relationship with the patient. This practice style does not encourage patient participation and raises issues of appropriate style, because it has been shown that patient participation increases functional outcomes (Henbest & Stewart, 1990; Kaplan, Greenfield, & Ware, 1985).

The changes in health care and the way that occupational therapy services are delivered are demanding an increased focus on accountability, restricted costs, and achieving outcomes. These services are provided in a context of consumers demanding increased involvement in decision making about health care practices. All of these issues have led to an increased focus on client involvement in occupational therapy services; that is, client-centred practice.

WHAT IS CLIENT-CENTRED OCCUPATIONAL THERAPY?

Client-centred practice has been defined as "an approach to service which embraces a philosophy of respect for, and partnership with, people receiving services" (Law, Baptiste, & Mills, 1995, p. 253). Although client-centredness has been part of the Canadian occupational therapy philosophy since the early 1980s, the definition proposed by Law et al. was the first formal definition of client-centred occupational therapy practice. Guidelines for the practice of client-centred occupational therapy in Canada define client-centred practice as

> *"collaborative approaches aimed at enabling occupation with clients who may be individuals, groups, agencies, governments, corporations or others. Occupational therapists demonstrate respect for clients, involve clients in decision making, advocate with and for clients in meeting clients' needs, and otherwise recognize clients' experience and knowledge" (Canadian Association of Occupational Therapists, 1997, p. 49).*

In occupational therapy, Canadian occupational therapists have been leaders in defining and discussing the practice of client-centred occupational therapy since the early 1980s. There has been much discussion in the Canadian occupational therapy literature about the involvement of clients in the therapy intervention process and how it can be facilitated in practice. Along with increasing emphasis on client-centred practice, the role of spirituality in practice has been emphasized. This focus on people receiving occupational therapy services finding meaning in everyday occupations has also been highlighted by studies of clinical reasoning funded by the American Occupational Therapy Association and the American Occupational Therapy Foundation. For example, Schwartz (1991) discussed the need for occupational therapists to understand a person's story of his or her life and what occupations he or she finds meaningful. Mattingly (1991) demonstrated in her studies of clinical reasoning that occupational therapists use narrative reasoning to help them understand people's values and desires for daily living.

Chewning and Sleath (1996) have contrasted intervention approaches using a medical model with a collaborative client-centred model. A medical model places an emphasis on a person's clinical status as defined by the service provider, patient education to ensure that the person complies with treatment, and outcomes as evaluated by the service provider. In contrast, in a client-centred collaborative model, the person receiving intervention defines the priorities together with the service provider, education focuses on increasing the person's self-management abilities, and both the client and provider evaluate outcomes.

Matheis-Kraft, George, Olinger, and York (1990) have defined the goal of health care in which people are full participants as "the goal of the patient-centred philosophy is to create a caring, dignified and empowering environment in which patients truly direct the course of their care and call upon their inner resources to speed the healing process" (p. 128).

HISTORICAL ROOTS OF CLIENT-CENTRED PRACTICE

The use of the term client-centred practice began with Carl Rogers. In his book, *The Clinical Treatment of the Problem Child* (Rogers, 1939), Rogers described a practice that was nondirective and focused on concerns as expressed by the client receiving the service. One of the key values of client-centred practice described by Rogers is a recognition of a person's unique cultural values. For example, Rogers stated, "Mostly deeply of all, it is built upon close, intimate and specific observations of man's behaviour in a relationship, observations which it is believed transcend to some degree the limitations or influences of a given culture" (Rogers, 1951, p. 5). Rogers believed that people receiving service are very capable of playing an active role in defining and solving problems.

The role of the therapist, according to Rogers, is to facilitate problem solving through stimulating the person's desire and ability to understand problems and propose solutions that are appropriate for his or her life. The theoretical constructs underpinning client-centred interactions evolved from learning theory and ideas about the self and the dynamics of interpersonal relationships (Rogers, 1951). One of the key features of client-centred therapy is the nondirectiveness of the therapist. Rogers did not believe that a therapist was more of an expert than the client. In fact, he stated that directive therapy was problematic because "the directive viewpoint places a high value on social conformity and the right of the more able to direct the less able" (Rogers, 1942, pp. 126-127). Therapists or counselors are most effective, in Rogers' view, when they are comfortable with their personal values and able to work with a client using a nonjudgmental approach. They recognize the client's need for growth and development and are open in sharing knowledge and providing relevant information to help the client solve his or her issues.

Rogers cautioned against placing too great an emphasis on therapeutic methods, as he felt that this got in the way of the counselor enabling the client to discover solutions. The danger in therapy focused on techniques and methods is that the client will be controlled. Another key characteristic of client-centred therapy as developed by Rogers was its phenomenological nature (Cain, 1990). An important assumption arising from this characteristic is that clients are the best individuals to describe their experiences and their reality. Because of this, it is important for therapists to spend enough time and listen to be able to learn about the client's life experiences.

In a client-centred approach, therapists acknowledge the differences of individuals. However, Rogers did not make specific suggestions about how to approach such diversities within practice. "A paradox of the client-centred approach is that it acknowledges and values the uniqueness of persons, it does not specify how the differences in clients might affect therapeutic practice" (Cain, 1990, p. 93). Cain goes on to state that for some individuals who have difficulty in reflecting on their experience, a more structured form of client-centred therapy may be appropriate.

One of the difficulties with client-centred therapy is its lack of specific methodologies. Rogers did not apologize for this; in fact, he stated, "The picture is one of fluid changes in a general approach to problems of human relationships, rather than a situation in which some relatively rigid technique is more or less mechanically applied" (Rogers, 1951, p. 6). Szasz and Hollender (1956) state that the key characteristics of client-centred approaches include respect for individuals and a focus on enabling clients to direct solutions to their stated issues. A client-centred approach focuses on facilitating people to provide the source of solution for their own problems rather than providing them with specific advice or telling them what to do. A client-centred approach is inherently optimistic, believing that all people are capable of making decisions about their daily lives (Bernard, 1995).

There have been criticisms of the client-centred approach. It has been stated that the client-centred emphasis on individuals and their inherent worth and their experience of problems ignores our common humanity and the fact that many of us encounter problems that are similar (Bernard, 1995). Rogers also does not provide suggestions about the best therapy approach in situations where people are not motivated or do not wish to change. May (1983) criticizes Rogers' approach for being overly optimistic and ignoring the fact that some people are truly evil.

In describing the historical underpinnings of client-centred practice, it is important to consider the historical roots of rehabilitation. The development of rehabilitation came during and immediately after the first World War. Rehabilitation continued to grow into the 1930s when the Depression halted its growth. Berkowitz (1989) states that rehabilitation reached a new maturity during and after the second World War, about the time that Rogers was developing his client-centred approach. The differences between the rehabilitation approach during the 1940s and 1950s and Rogers' client-centred therapy are quite dramatic. While Rogers' client-centred approach was nondirective and valued people's individuality and experiences, the rehabilitation approach focused on the use of a medical model in which a rehabilitation diagnosis was made, and specific treatment techniques were prescribed to be followed by therapists and patients. Although a team approach was emphasized from the beginning of rehabilitation medicine, the physician was clearly the de facto leader of the team. It was not until the past two decades that people with disabilities rose up in protest to standard methods of rehabilitation and discrimination within our society (Gliedman & Roth, 1980). At the same time as all consumers were demanding more participation and control over societal issues, people with disabilities demanded more control over rehabilitation practices.

THE WORDS WE USE TO DESCRIBE THIS APPROACH TO PRACTICE

During the past decade, there have been many terms used to describe concepts centred on people being partners in health care. These terms include client-centred, client-driven, patient-centred, and patient-focused care. Gage (1995) provides a thorough discussion of these models of care. She quite rightly states that many of the concepts that are attributed to each term are very similar. Systems of care appear to be described as patient-centred or patient-focused if they emanate from an institution or hospital setting, where people are primarily known as patients. When people are receiving services outside of a hospital, or from a particular health discipline such as occupational therapy or social work, they tend to be referred to as clients.

Key differences in the descriptions seem to be through the use of the words centred, focused, or driven. Gage (1995) argues that the preferred practice term should be client-driven, to describe a practice in which clients make decisions about the focus of therapy and are empowered to achieve solutions. Her description of client-centred therapy, as one can see, is virtually identical to Rogers' description of the client-centred approach. The difficulty with the term client-centred is that it has been used by institutions and writers to describe approaches that may not be conceptually consistent with Rogers' original ideas. In pediatric rehabilitation, the description of a family-centred partnership between families and service providers and the family leading the decision-making process is consistent with the original concepts put forth by Rogers (Gage, 1995). In describing models of client-driven approaches, Gage describes the Planetree model of health care and the work by the Picker-Commonwealth program. It is interesting, however, to note that articles describing the Planetree model are key-worded under patient-centred care and the Picker-Commonwealth program is also labeled patient-centred care. There appears to be a clearer distinction between client-centred or client-driven care, and client- or patient-focused care. Patient-focused care appears to be based largely on a model of organizational change that focuses activities within an institution specifically on the patient, in order to streamline activities and make them more efficient and less costly (Gage, 1995).

In reviewing this dilemma about terminology, it is clear there is a need for specific definitions of the concepts inherent with each term. It appears that there are many situations in which the terms family-centred, patient-centred, or client-centred practice are very similar to that described as client-driven practice. The descriptions of client-centred practice espouse the same principles as Rogers did originally in describing a client-centred approach. It would, therefore, seem most appropriate to use terminology that is consistent with Rogers' approach in describing the concepts and use his preferred terminology of client-centred.

IMPORTANT CONCEPTS OF CLIENT-CENTRED PRACTICE

Until recently, the important concepts that define client-centred occupational therapy have not been outlined in detail in the occupational therapy literature. While issues of client motivation, client-therapist communication, and client involvement in the therapy process have been discussed, Law, Baptiste, and Mills (1995) were the first authors to discuss key concepts of client-centred occupational therapy and the implications of these for practice. In 1997, the Canadian Association of Occupational Therapists published a book to describe the process of enabling occupation and included a discussion of 10 important principles of client-centred occupational therapy (Canadian Association of Occupational Therapists, 1997). The key concepts of client-centred occupational therapy described by Law, Baptiste, and Mills (1995) and by the Canadian Association of Occupational Therapists (1997) are outlined in Table 1-1.

In other areas of the health care system, such as hospital-based care and services for children, the concepts of patient-centred care and family-centred care/service have been outlined in detail. For example, the Picker-Commonwealth Program for Patient-Centred Care has developed seven dimensions of patient-centred care, based on research with more than 6,000 patients and 2,000 family members (Gerteis, Edgman-Levitan, Daley, & Delbanco, 1993). Also in the hospital-based sector, Planetree has developed a model of hospital-based care for its hospital units (Blank, Horowitz, & Matza, 1995). Through the process of developing a model unit for a hospital in New York, Planetree incorporated a number of key concepts of patient care in the delivery of hospital-based services. The key concepts from the Picker-Commonwealth and the Planetree models are also outlined in Table 1-1.

Some of the earliest and most comprehensive work to define concepts of how care is provided has been coordinated through the Association for the Care of Children's Health (ACCH) in Bethesda, Md. The passage of the Education for All Handicapped Children Act, or UJA Public Law-142 mandated that parents be involved in setting goals for services for their children. In 1986, Public Law-457 extended these ideas and stated that the whole family should be involved in the service process and make decisions on goals and services for their children. The ACCH defined eight dimensions of family-centred care (Shelton, Jeppson, & Johnson, 1987) (see Table 1-1). In Canada, the Neurodevelopmental Clinical Research Unit at McMaster University, in partnership with the Ontario Association of Children's Rehabilitation Services, have developed a conceptual framework for family-centred service (Rosenbaum, King, Law, King, & Evans, in press). This conceptual framework outlines the basic assumptions, guiding principles and important ser-

Table 1-1
Concepts of Client-Centred Practice

Law, Baptiste & Mills (1995)	Blank, Horowitz & Matza (1995)	Gerteis, Edgman-Levitan, Daley & Delbanco (1993)	Rosenbaum, King, Law, King & Evans (in press)	Association for the Care of Children's Health (1987)	CAOT (1997)
• client autonomy and choice • respect for diversity • partnership and responsibility • enablement • contextual congruence • accessibility and flexibility	• patient is an active participant in care • patient participation in decision-making • design of hospital environment to enhance comfort • family involvement • provide information in accessible ways; emphasize communication	• respect for patients' values, preferences and needs • care coordination and integration • provision of information, education; emphasis on communication • provide physical comfort • provide emotional support • involve family and friends in care process • continuity of care; assist in transition to community and/or other services	• encourage parent decision-making • families decide level of involvement • parents have ultimate responsibility for their children • respect for families and their diversity • consider needs of all family members • encourage use of community supports • encourage involvement of all family members • provide individualized service • collaboration • accessibility	• family is the constant in the child's life • parent-professional collaboration • sharing of information • comprehensive policies/programs that meet families' needs • recognition of family strengths, individuality; respect for different methods of coping • understanding and incorporation of the developmental needs of children, adolescents and families • encourage parent-to-parent support • flexible, accessible, responsive health care delivery systems	• listen to client values, meaning and choice • help clients see what might be possible • provide support for client success, but also to risk • respect clients' coping & strengths • facilitate client identification of needs and meaningful outcomes • facilitate client participation in all aspects of occupational therapy service • provide information • do not overwhelm clients with bureaucracy • emphasize open communication

vice provider behaviours that make up a family-centred service approach to providing service.

A review of the six frameworks in Table 1-1 reveals that, while there are some differences in emphasis, there are several common ideas within all frameworks that can be used to define client-centred practice for occupational therapists (Table 1-2).

Table 1-2
Concepts of Client-Centred Practice Common to all Models

- Respect for clients and their families, and the choices they make.
- Clients and families have the ultimate responsibility for decisions about daily occupations and occupational therapy services.
- Provision of information, physical comfort, and emotional support. Emphasis on person-centred communication.
- Facilitation of client participation in all aspects of occupational therapy service.
- Flexible, individualized occupational therapy service delivery.
- Enabling clients to solve occupational performance issues.
- Focus on the person-environment-occupation relationship.

- All client-centred, patient-centred, and family-centred frameworks begin by emphasizing the need for respect for clients and their families. Clients of occupational therapy come from many different backgrounds, have encountered different life experiences, and have made choices regarding occupation that are unique to them and the situation in which they live. Clients have developed styles of coping with the challenges that they encounter in daily living on a day-to-day basis. A fundamental concept of client-centred occupational therapy is that therapists show respect for the choices that clients have made, choices that they will make, and their personal methods of coping.

Respect for clients and their families, and the choices they make

Susan is experiencing difficulties with occupation due to back pain from a work injury. She is currently receiving a disability pension. Susan is unable to drive, yet she chooses to live in a rural setting that is isolated from public transportation, and community services. The occupational performance areas identified by Susan as her needs for occupational therapy include: (1) environmental set up for loading wood into the stove to maintain heat; (2) environmental layout for laundry area; (3) access transportation when required. While information is provid ed regarding other living arrangements that would conserve energy and promote community involvement, Susan's value of maintaining her rural lifestyle is respected.

Mary is a senior living in a remote setting. She has had an above knee amputation and prosthesis for many years, and recently developed tendinitis in her shoulder. Her bedroom is located upstairs. Currently, she transfers for her hygiene by crawling to the bathroom, and hoisting herself up on the toilet or over the high wall of her old fashioned bathtub. Observation by the occupational therapist notes that this method of doing transfers is extremely strenuous, requiring excessive upper body strength, and compromising her shoulder with tendinitis. Mary does not want to consider any option other than using her old fashioned bathtub. Through occupational therapy intervention, her home environment is modified to eliminate the need for crawling and floor-to-standing transfers. Transfer heights are all raised, and rest stations positioned where dressing/undressing is needed. A transfer method is designed and taught to Mary that allows her safe access to the old fashioned tub. Although this method is more difficult than other strategies explored, the extra effort/difficulty is worth the benefit of maintaining her use of her bathtub.

- Once respect is shown for the diverse nature of clients and their issues, it is obvious that clients and families have the ultimate responsibility for decisions about their daily occupations and the occupational therapy services they receive. Clients hold the most important information about their needs and should be encouraged to make choices and to define the occupational performance issues for which they require occupational therapy intervention. How often does this occur in current occupational therapy practice? Northen et al. (1995) found that while therapists did involve clients in the goal-setting process, less than 50% of the goal-setting criteria were used during these initial occupational therapy sessions. Neistadt and Seymour (1995) found that when more formal methods are used to gain knowledge about clients' priorities, intervention focuses more on functional activities than on remedial approaches focused on improving performance components.

Clients and families have the ultimate responsibility for decisions about daily occupations and occupational therapy services

Samantha is a 70 year old woman who recently had a stroke and was discharged home. Her husband prefers to provide assistance with dressing and bathing. Samantha and her husband both agree that this is the best use of both of their time rather than focusing on independence that tires her out, or worries him. The occupational therapist works within this framework providing strategies that allow for a safe environment. She also facilitates efficient movement patterns while the husband is assisting the wife, without imposing the value of "independence at all costs" upon their daily routine.

An occupational therapist is working with a 72 year old man in a nursing home. He had a stroke that has resulted in compromised judgment and occasional impulsivity, in addition to ataxia and weakness that make unsupervised transfers unsafe. He is able to walk with the assistance of one person, using a walker. However, he has been unable to progress to walking by himself and becomes frustrated when having to wait for assistance. His family requested occupational therapy for a wheelchair prescription. The client is upset about using a wheelchair, but is agreeable since his main goal is to leave the dining room independently, and not have to wait 30 minutes for everyone to leave the dining room in order. Once the occupational therapist provided the appropriate equipment to allow the client to be independent, the risk of him transferring back to bed unsupervised and unsafely was introduced, as he could leave the dining room on his own. This was difficult for the nursing home to accept initially. The occupational therapist was able to successfully facilitate an agreement for the nursing home staff to accept that the family was willing to assume the increased risk of falling in order to have the client able to leave the dining room on his own free will. Environmental strategies were put into place to minimize the risk as much as possible.

- Provision of physical comfort, emotional support, information to enable decision making, and an emphasis on communication are commonly cited in all of the frameworks for client-centred practice. Clients need to feel comfortable in the occupational therapy setting, whether it is hospital-based or in the community. Information about their occupational performance issues and potential solutions, if given in an understandable way, helps clients to make decisions about the intervention process. Kalmanson and Seligman (1992), in discussing interventions for young children, state that "the success of all interventions will rest on the quality of provider-family relationships, even when the relationship itself is not the focus of the intervention"

(p. 48). The relationship and interactions between clients and occupational therapists deserve much more attention than they have received in the past. An open, caring relationship in which the occupational therapist hears the story that the person has to tell and listens to the description of his or her needs can only enhance the ability of the person and therapist to work together to solve occupational performance issues. Kasch and Knutson (1985) make a distinction between two types of speech that are used in professional services. They believe that "position-centred speech" is based on professionals' adherence to certain norms of behaviour and a need to ensure that people behave according to expectations and that rules are followed. Some examples of position-centred speech they cite include the following: "You should start showing up for your appointment on time"; "We are trying everything possible to help..."; "I think it's important that you..." (p. 53). In contrast, they state that "person-centred speech" is more individualized, with the service provider focusing on the individual needs of the client at that particular time. Examples of person-centred speech cited by Kasch and Knutson include the following: "Even if your sore throat feels much better in 3 or 4 days, it is important that you take the full 10 days of medication"; "The 10-day treatment of medication gives you the best protection against developing a complication" (p. 54).

Provision of information, physical comfort, and emotional support. Emphasis on person-centred communication

---

A 37 year old young man with multiple sclerosis is referred to occupational therapy. His condition is deteriorating, resulting in progressive quadriplegia. The man's physician has suggested to the client and his family that his condition is palliative. For the man and his family, physical comfort during the night is a concern, as his breathing becomes very difficult and his chest is difficult to clear. To achieve these goals, the use of a hoyer lift for his wife to use with him, and the introduction of a hospital bed for elevation at night to assist with breathing, is suggested. These substantial changes to their household are not forced upon the couple, but rather emotional support, information regarding the rationale for the recommendations, and open communication regarding the impact on sleeping arrangements for their relationship are explored. The couple decide to go ahead with the changes, invest in a single bed to be placed beside the hospital bed, and learn the use of the hoyer lift for times of the day when fatigue prevents a safe unassisted transfer.

- Client participation to facilitate a collaborative partnership between clients and occupational therapists is another fundamental concept of client-centred practice. The development of a partnership between clients and occupational therapists is facilitated by a conscious shift of power from the therapist to the client. This shift in power occurs when it is the client who identifies the occupational performance issues for occupational therapy intervention, participates actively in decisions about the intervention focus, and defines the outcomes of occupational therapy service. There are different levels of client participation in service provider-client interactions. Szasz and Hollender (1956) defined three models on a continuum of participation, ranging from client-dependent to client-cooperative to mutual participation. The goal of client-centred occupational therapy is to ensure that the relationship between the therapist and client is one of mutual participation. Pesznecker, Zerwekh, and Horn (1989) emphasize the need for clients and service providers to develop a mutual participation relationship. This has been defined as a relationship "in which the provider and client have approximately equal power in the relationship, are mutually interdependent, and engage in activities that will in some ways be satisfying to each other" (p. 197).

Facilitation of client participation in all aspects of occupational therapy service

A 45 year old woman who lives alone has been referred to occupational therapy. She has had depression for many years and is currently experiencing difficulty maintaining cleanliness of her apartment, and organizing household bills. She is afraid that she will not be able to continue to live on her own. Her goal for occupational therapy intervention is to be able to continue to live in her own apartment. From the initial visit, the client is engaged in planning the occupational therapy services, involved in deciding the acceptable visit frequency, and setting objectives toward progress that could be expected across the visits. The occupational therapist needs to be flexible with her schedule to adapt to the emotional difficulties that the client has on various days. In the end, the goals of having an organized system for coping with household management are in place, and drawn up by the client.

• All frameworks of client-centred, family-centred, or patient-centred care focus on the way in which health care delivery systems are structured. To be client-centred, a service system must be flexible so that the individualized needs of the client and his or her family are considered in every aspect of service provision. Services are accessible and coordinated so that clients understand the process and can easily participate in service delivery. All of the frameworks that were reviewed emphasize the need to ensure that the health system bureaucracy does not overwhelm clients and their families.

Flexible, individualized occupational therapy service delivery

Bill has been admitted to the rehabilitation floor in a general hospital. He has a 10 year history of advanced peripheral neuropathy in the lower extremities that require the use of metal leg braces bilaterally, and extensive use of a rollator walker. He was admitted to hospital due to a fractured humerus from falling when an elevator door closed too quickly. Using the Canadian Occupational Performance Measure, the therapist finds that Bill's main goal is to return living alone with Home Care Support. His concerns include walking, using the fractured arm for washing and dressing, and toilet transfers. Initially, therapy focuses on gentle mobilization of the arm, gradually introducing basic aspects of hygiene and dressing. As partial weight bearing on the impaired arm through the walker is permitted, daily living tasks are advanced. Factors to be considered include seat height, floor covering surface, and hand hold placement to accurately simulate the home environment. Training for night time transfers is needed because he does not wear braces at night. It is essential that the client define many issues regarding the transfer method that will work within his home environment. The control that Bill exerts during the therapy process is labeled by some staff as manipulative and demanding. However, respecting the environmental context in which the client had to be prepared to function is essential to developing the skills and personal confidence for a safe return home. A home visit is completed to ensure that Bill had achieved adequate independence to return to living alone. Strategies for coping with the elevator were reviewed and followed up by Home Care in the community.

A 5 year old girl with hemiplegia (cerebral palsy) is referred for a fine motor assessment/intervention. The typical approach to this referral would be to complete a battery of fine motor and perceptual motor assessments. However, upon the first visit to the school, and in talking wih her parents, it is found that the main concerns in the classroom are: (1) accessing the bathroom through a heavy door; and (2) waiting for the bus after school (made difficult because of a short attention span). It is determined that the environmental consultation regarding these issues is a priority over an assessment battery, despite the original referral. This is clarified with the referring agency, and intervention time focuses on the school's and parents' primary concerns first.

- A focus on enabling and facilitating client involvement and client-defined outcomes is inherent in client-centred occupational therapy. The therapist is not the expert who provides solutions to occupational performance problems. In a client-centred approach, the therapist is a facilitator working to enable the client to generate and implement solutions. In the process of solving one occupational performance problem, clients gain skills that enable them to resolve future issues that they may encounter in performing daily occupations.

Enabling clients to solve occupational performance issues

A 28 year old man has quadriplegia from a spinal cord injury, and has been experiencing upper back pain for one year. He is referred to occupational therapy for the prescription of a wheelchair. He has been able to push a rigid lightweight manual wheelchair since his accident, but this past year, his mobility has been limited by the back pain. The pain is worst when propelling the wheelchair, and muscle spasms are also jeopardizing his safety with independent transfers. The primary issue for the client is whether to continue using a manual wheelchair and different positioning, or to change to a power wheelchair to minimize strain on the upper torso and hopefully, help to control his pain. The client is not certain what to do, and wants the therapist to make this decision. Instead of making a recommendation, the therapist works with the client so that he is able to explore various mobility options. After this process, he is able to come to a decision that the use of power mobility will significantly improve the quality of his daily living.

- A unique concept within client-centred occupational therapy is the acknowledgment that clients are not divorced from the environments and community in which they live, work, and play. Whether this is labeled as contextual congruence, use of community supports, continuity of care, or transition issues, the recognition that clients' roles and lives within a larger community context need to be considered in all aspects of service delivery is important. We know, from person-environment behaviour theories, that environments can have either a facilitating or constraining effect on a person's roles and their daily occupations (Law, Cooper, Stewart, Letts, Rigby, & Strong, 1994). Emerging models of practice in occupational therapy emphasize the person-environment-occupation relationship and the ability of occupational therapy intervention to focus on changing the environment to facilitate occupational performance (Law, Cooper, Strong, Stewart, Rigby, & Letts, 1997).

> **Focus on the person environment occupational relationship**
>
> Mark is a 42 year old young man who has acquired brain injury following a car accident. He is referred to occupational therapy two years post injury due to difficulties he was experiencing in completing job trials for a vocational assessment program. Mark's cognitive difficulties resulting from the brain injury include memory problems, difficulties with names and word finding, difficulty with problem solving through new social situations, poor reading comprehension, and stress related headaches. He is also frustrated because he wants to drive again. His strengths include automatic social skills, high motivation and work ethic, and physical strength/coordination. The job trials that are causing problems are in the shipping and receiving department of two busy stores, where he stocks shelves and relates to customers when necessary. His entire previous work experience was focused on construction work, working extensively on automobiles, or driving heavy machinery. Occupational therapy intervention focuses on: (1) working with Mark to develop strategies for the job trial; this is successful but difficult for him as the job setting is entirely unrelated to anything he had done previously; (2) consulting with the job trial coordinator searching for an environment that will capitalize on Mark's strengths and past experience; and (3) making appropriate contacts to enable Mark to complete an assessment for driving license reinstatement that has been held up unnecessarily. By addressing the environment in which the client is required to work, Mark is able to successfully complete a job trial in a garage setting and receive his license so he could legally move vehicles around the parking lot. Increasing Mark's coping strategies is not enough. The fit between Mark, his work environment, and the occupation needs to be addressed to ensure successful outcomes after intervention.

THE CHALLENGES OF CLIENT-CENTRED OCCUPATIONAL THERAPY

There are many challenges as occupational therapists and clients work together to implement client-centred occupational therapy practice. As we reframe the occupational therapy practice process to enable clients to identify and solve occupational performance issues, changes are required to the way in which therapists have always practiced. In a discussion of ethical issues in family-centred early intervention, Sokoly and Dokecki (1992) state that there is a need for all professionals to "question the accepted ways of doing things" (p. 25). Our expectations for ourselves in a client-centred practice will change. Client-centred occupational therapists will develop into reflective practitioners (Schon, 1983), working together with clients in a flexible manner to solve occupational performance problems. The ability to work together with clients to ensure a common understanding of the clients' needs and goals from occupational therapy is a key to ensuring strong, effective service provider-client relationships.

While many have written about the challenges of implementing client and family-centred service, there have been a few studies that have investigated these issues. A recent study using in-depth interviews with 13 service providers in children s rehabilitation centres found that the process of change in implementing family-centred service was dynamic, with change being constant and a sense that the end was not in sight (Law, Brown, Barnes, King, Rosenbaum, & King, 1997). Time and resources were identified as the most significant challenges in implementing a family-centred service. The way in which some services were structured led to inherent organizational barriers that limited interaction and partnership between families and service providers. The physical environment of a facility can enhance the welcoming feeling that families and clients have when they come for service. On the other hand, high noise levels, crowded space, or lack of space to meet cause increased problems. Families and clients will differ in how much they want to participate in a partnership. Each client comes with different experiences and levels of confidence. In this way, client-centred service is challenging, both for the client and the occupational therapist. For clients who are not familiar with client-centred service, negotiation about service provision may be difficult.

The implementation of client-centred occupational therapy takes time. It is important that occupational therapists understand their own beliefs and values, as well as develop new skills in areas such as negotiation. There may be occasions when occupational therapists are reluctant to ask clients what they desire, because they fear they may not be able to provide it. There is certainly a need for more information on a practical level to aid the implementation of client-centred occupational therapy.

REFERENCES

Berkowitz, E. D. (1989). Allocating resources for rehabilitation: A historical and ethical framework. *Social Sciences Quarterly, 70,* 40-52.

Bernard, P. (1995). Implications of client-centred counseling for nursing practice. *Nursing Times, 91,* 35-37.

Blank, A. E., Horowitz, S., & Matza, D. (1995). Quality with a human face? The Samuels Planetree model hospital unit. *Journal on Quality Improvement, 21,* 289-299.

Cain, D. J. (1990). Further thoughts about non-directiveness and client-centred therapy. *Person-Centered Review, 5,* 89-99.

Canadian Association of Occupational Therapists (1997). *Enabling occupation: An occupational therapy perspective.* Ottawa, ON: CAOT Publications ACE.

Chewning, B., & Sleath, B. (1996). Medication decision-making and management: A client-centred model. *Social Sciences and Medicine, 42,* 389-398.

Epp, H. (1986). *Achieving health for all: A framework for health promotion* (Report No. H39-102/1987E). Ottawa, ON: Health and Welfare Canada.

Gage, M. (1995). Re-engineering of health care: Opportunity or threat for occupational therapists? *Canadian Journal of Occupational Therapy, 62*(4), 197-207.

Gerteis, M., Edgman-Levitan, S., Daley, J., & Delbanco, T. L. (1993). *Through the patient's eyes: Understanding and promoting patient-centred care.* San Francisco: Jossey-Bass Publishers.

Gliedman, J., & Roth, W. (1980). *The unexpected minority: Handicapped children in America.* New York: Harcourt Brace Jovanovich.

Greenfield, S., Kaplan, S.H., & Ware, J.E. (1985). Expanding patient involvement in care: Effects on patient outcomes. *Annals of Internal Medicine, 102,* 520-528.

Haiman, S. (1995). Dilemmas in professional collaboration with consumers. *Journal of Psychiatric Services, 46,* 443-445.

Henbest, R. J., & Stewart, M. (1990). Patient-centredness in the consultation. II: Does it really make a difference? *Family Practice, 7,* 28-33.

Johnson, R. (1993). Attitudes don't just hang in the air...Disabled people's perceptions of physiotherapists. *Physiotherapy, 79*, 619-626.

Kalmanson, B., & Seligman, S. (1992). Family-provider relationships: The basis of all interventions. *Infants & Young Children, 4*(4), 46-52.

Kasch, C. R., & Knutson, K. (1985). Patient compliance and interpersonal style: Implications for practice and research. *Journal of Nurse Practitioner*, March, 52-54.

Law, M., Baptiste, S., & Mills, J. (1995). Client-centred practice: What does it mean and does it make a difference? *Canadian Journal of Occupational Therapy, 62*, 250-257.

Law, M., Brown, S., Barnes, S., King, G., Rosenbaum, P., & King, S. (1997). *Implementing family-centred service in Ontario at children's rehabilitation centres.* Hamilton, ON: Neurodevelopmental Clinical Research Unit, McMaster University.

Law, M., Cooper, B., Strong, S., Stewart, D., Rigby, P., & Letts, L. (1997). A theoretical context for the practice of occupational therapy. In C. Christensen & C. Baum (Eds.). *Occupational therapy achieving human performance needs in daily living (2nd ed.).* Thorofare, NJ: SLACK Incorporated.

Law, M., Cooper, B., Stewart, D., Letts, L., Rigby, P., & Strong, S. (1994). Person-environment relations. *Work, 4*, 228-238.

Matheis-Kraft, C., George, S., Olinger, M. J., & York, L. (1990). Patient-driven health care works. *Nursing Management, 21*, 124-128.

Mattingly, C. (1991). The narrative nature of clinical reasoning. *American Journal of Occupational Therapy, 45*, 998-1005.

May, R. (1983). The problem of evil: An open letter to Carl Rogers. *Journal of Humanistic Psychology, 122*, 10-21.

Moorehead, R., & Winefield, H. (1991). Teaching counselling skills to fourth year medical students: A dilemma concerning goals. *Family Practice, 8*, 343-346.

Neistadt, M. E., & Seymour, S. T. (1995). Treatment activity preferences of occupational therapists in adult physical dysfunction settings. *American Journal of Occupational Therapy, 49*, 437-443.

Neistadt, M. E. (1995). Methods of assessing clients' priorities: A survey of adult physical dysfunction settings. *American Journal of Occupational Therapy, 49*, 428-436.

Northen, J. G., Rust, D. M., Nelson, C. E., & Watts, J. H. (1995). Involvement of adult rehabilitation patients in setting occupational therapy goals. *American Journal of Occupational Therapy, 49*, 214-220.

Pesznecker, B. L., Zerwekh, J. V., & Horn, B. J. (1989). The mutual-participation relationship: Key to facilitating self-care practices in clients and families. *Public Health Nursing, 6*, 197-203.

Rogers, C. R. (1939). *The clinical treatment of the problem child.* Boston: Houghton-Mifflin.

Rogers, C. R. (1942). *Counselling and psychotherapy.* Boston: Houghton-Mifflin.

Rogers, C. R. (1951). *Client-centred therapy.* Boston: Houghton-Mifflin.

Rosenbaum, P., King, S., Law, M., King, G., & Evans, J. (In press). Family-centred service: A conceptual framework and research review. *Physical & Occupational Therapy in Pediatrics.*

Schon, D. (1983). *The reflective practitioner.* San Francisco: Jossey-Bass Publishers.

Schwartz, K. B. (1991). Clinical reasoning and new ideas on intelligence: Implications for teaching and learning. *American Journal of Occupational Therapy, 45*, 1033-1037.

Shelton, T. L., Jeppson, E. S., & Johnson, B. H. (1987). *Underlining family-centred care for children with special health care needs.* Washington, DC: Association for the Care of Children's Health.

Sokoly, M. M., & Dokecki, P. R. (1992). Ethical perspectives on family-centred early intervention. Infants & *Young Children, 4*(4), 23-32.

Swanson, L. (1997) Canadian farmers with disabilities: Experts in the fields. *Abilities, 30*, 50-51.

Szasz, T. A., & Hollender, M. H. (1956). A contribution to the philosophy of medicine: The basic models of the doctor-patient relationship. *Archives of Internal Medicine, 97*, 585-592.

chapter

DOES CLIENT-CENTRED PRACTICE MAKE A DIFFERENCE?

MARY LAW, PHD, OT(C)

People receiving occupational therapy services want to know and often assume that the intervention that they receive will make a difference to their function and quality of life. Health care payers are also demanding evidence to support the effectiveness of occupational therapy interventions. An occupational therapy practice based on evidence of effectiveness will ensure that our clients receive best quality service, and in the end will save costs if functional outcomes are improved.

There are two dimensions to evidence-based occupational therapy: the specific intervention approach used and how service is delivered. The specific intervention approach is determined after an analysis of the person-environment-occupation relationship for each individual. Once problems in occupational performance have been identified by the client, the most appropriate theoretical intervention approach is chosen for the identified performance issues. Examples of these intervention approaches include intervention based on the Canadian Model of Occupational Performance (Canadian Association of Occupational Therapists, 1997), the Model of Human Occupation (Kielhofner, 1995), environmental modification (Law, Cooper, Strong, Stewart, Rigby, & Letts, 1996), or a cognitive behavioural approach. Evidence supporting the efficacy and effectiveness of intervention, or the "what" that occupational therapists do, is essential. Equally important is evidence of the "how" in terms of how occupational therapy services are delivered. This book outlines a method for the delivery of occupational therapy services called client-centred occupational therapy. It is important to review research evidence so that therapists will know whether client-centred occupational therapy (how service is delivered) makes a difference.

TYPES OF RESEARCH EVIDENCE

Research studies evaluating delivery of service range from single person testimonials to randomized clinical trials. Both qualitative and quantitative approaches to studying service delivery in occupational therapy and in other health professions have been utilized. The challenge for therapists is to determine the strength of the evidence reported within any particular study or across a series of studies.

Many authors have developed criteria for critically reviewing research completed using quantitative methods (Sackett, Haynes, Guyatt, & Tugwell, 1991; Law, 1987; Guyatt, Sackett, & Cook, 1993). Criteria used by these authors include study design, similarity between groups within the study, biases present, reliability and validity of outcome measures, sampling, statistical and clinical significance, size of the treatment effect, completeness of follow-up, precision of the treatment effect, and applicability of results to the reader's practice. Groups such as the Cochrane Collaboration, an international network for the review of evidence-based practice (Huston, 1996), support the completion of systmatic reviews in many areas of health care. When reviews of evidence are completed, t   overall results of the review can be summarized using meta-analysis and/or levels of evi   nce (Sackett, 1993).

Reviews of research using qualitative methods have focused on issues of design, purpose of the study, sampling, evidence of triangulation, methods of analysis, trustworthiness of the data and findings, use of negative case analysis, and checking for all alternative explanations for the findings (Lincoln & Guba, 1985; Patton, 1990; Forchuck & Roberts, 1993).

RESEARCH ON CLIENT-CENTRED PRACTICE

Before writing this chapter, a review of the literature studying client-centred practice was completed using the key terms client-centred, patient-centred, patient-focused, and family-centred service. All major health and psychological computer indices were searched from 1980 to 1997. As well, the bibliographies of pertinent research studies were searched for further evidence. The literature search was not confined to occupational therapy practice, but included all aspects of health care service delivery.

The research studies that were reviewed are clustered according to the primary outcomes that were investigated: adherence to intervention recommendations, client satisfaction, and functional outcome. The results of the research review will be described according to these three areas.

ADHERENCE TO INTERVENTION RECOMMENDATIONS

In a study using qualitative methods of participant observation and in-depth interviews, Avis (1994) observed 12 people within a surgical unit and interviewed 10 following surgery to examine their experiences with participation. Within this surgical setting, people expected to be told what to do and did not ask many questions. They often sought information from friends and family, but were not proactive in asking questions of health professionals. Avis contends that lack of knowledge by people coming to a surgery may significantly impact their ability to participate and ask questions. Patients may develop an "instrumental" approach to surgery, treating it as work in order to reconcile the difference in power status between themselves and health professionals. Power differentials and poor communication were the most important factors to diminish the ability of people to participate in this health care experience.

King, King, and Rosenbaum (1996) reviewed studies of the relationship between aspects of caregiving, information exchange, support and partnership, and their effect on client satisfaction, adherence, and stress. From their review of the evidence of caregiving and client adherence, King, King, and Rosenbaum state that providing service that supports the client and is respectful has been shown to be significantly associated with increased adherence to intervention recommendations. There is a need for further research to investigate other aspects of service delivery, such as providing information and working in partnership with clients to determine the effect of these characteristics on adherence in rehabilitation practice.

CLIENT SATISFACTION

King, Rosenbaum, and King (1996) found a significant relationship between giving of information, partnership, supportive and respectful care, and parent satisfaction with children's rehabilitation services. Satisfaction is determined more by the communication and the way in which a health professional conducts an encounter than by the content of what takes place. Being treated with respect and receiving information that will help decision making has been shown in a number of studies to increase client satisfaction (Doyle & Ware, 1977; Calnan, Katsouyiannopoulos, Ovcharov, Prokhorskas, Ramic, & Williams, 1994; Ben-Sira, 1976; Wasserman, Inui, Barriatua, Carter, & Lippincott, 1984).

A study by Caro and Derevensky (1991) indicated that 16 parents whose children received a family-focused, home-based intervention had very high degrees of satisfaction with the individualized nature of the program that was provided. A study by Kirkhart (1995) demonstrates improved client and physician satisfaction and decreased costs after implementation of a family-focused care delivery system emphasizing increased partnership and participation between health service providers and clients.

Abramson (1990) reviewed five studies of the discharge planning process. Results of these studies indicate that a client's degree of control has a significant effect on his or her satisfaction with the discharge planning process. Participation of clients in any decisions about relocation and discharge has been shown to decrease the negative outcomes of relocation.

Henbest and Fehrsen (1992) studied the applicability of patient-centredness in medical practice in a non-Western context, specifically among the poor in South Africa. Using a reliable and valid scale of patient-centredness, they found that the patient-centred nature varied significantly among five medical doctors and three nurse practitioners. The contents of the medical encounters were rated by masked reviewers for their patient-centred characteristics. A follow-up was completed with patients to determine their overall satisfaction with the medical encounter. Significantly higher levels of satisfaction and a belief that their symptoms had improved were noted for patients whose encounter scores were higher on the scale of patient-centred characteristics.

Using a prospective follow-up study, Henbest and Stewart (1990) audiotaped medical consultations for 73 people receiving service from family physicians. Independent ratings of the patient-centredness of the consultation were completed, as well as structured interviews with patients at the time of the consultation and 2 weeks later. There was a significant relationship between the patient-centred score for the medical encounter and patient satisfaction that their concerns had been heard and understood by the physician. On follow-up interview, 90% of the patients were quite satisfied with the encounter, and there was no significant association between the patient-centred score and patient satisfaction. As well, there was no significant association between the patient-centred score and symptom resolution at the 2-week follow-up. The authors state that the lack of significant association between the patient-centred encounter and satisfaction was likely influenced by the relatively small number of highly patient-centred encounters found in this study.

Dunst, Trivette, Boyd, and Brookfield (1994) have completed three studies comparing an expertise model to a direct guidance model and an empowerment model for service provision. The results of all studies indicate that the empowerment model, which encourages parent involvement and decision making, leads to an increased sense of control and satisfaction for parents.

In a study using both quantitative and qualitative data with 32 mothers of children with developmental problems, Marcenko & Smith (1992) found that a family-centred approach led to increased satisfaction of mothers, particularly related to information and advocacy services that were provided.

Stein and Jessop (1984, 1991) conducted a randomized controlled trial with 219 families of children with chronic illnesses. One group received a pediatric home-care program, while the other received standard care offered by their hospitals. The families who received the pediatric home-care program were significantly more satisfied with the services that they had received. As well, the children of these families showed significantly improved psychological adjustment. The functional status of the children in both groups was similar. In 1991, Stein and Jessop did a follow-up study of these groups and found that the children who had been in the pediatric home-care program continued to score significantly higher in terms of adjustment. They believe the aspects of the home-care program that led to these improved outcomes were the family-centred aspects of the program, which encouraged parents to make decisions about their children's care and to work in partnership with service providers.

Cleary, Edgman-Levitan, Roberts, Moloney, McMullen, Walker, and Delbanco (1991) interviewed 6,455 adults after discharge from 62 randomly-selected hospitals in the United States. Important areas of service provision that were rated by high percentages of patients as a problem included lack of the development of a trusting relationship with hospital staff, lack of information about the daily routine, lack of availability of the doctor to answer questions, and poor information related to discharge planning. Areas that were rated as being well done included explanation of tests and medications, staff trying to meet the patients' needs, and encouragement of family participation. There were significant differences according to health status, with sicker patients more likely to encounter problems in the way that they were treated.

Not all studies of client satisfaction show an increase after programs that emphasize information provision and partnership. For example, initial studies of the Planetree patient-centred model of care indicated that there were no significant differences in satisfaction between patients on a medical floor that was patient-centred compared to those on comparable standard floors. Nurses and nursing assistants, however, were significantly more satisfied with the patient-centred focus. The results of the patient satisfaction surveys did not take into account severity of illness, and this may have led to differences in these results when compared to other studies. A further complication that was encountered in this study was that close to 60% of those surveyed on the patient-centred unit had been transferred there from another unit in the hospital, so it is difficult to determine if they were discriminating between these two units when completing the patient satisfaction surveys.

FUNCTIONAL OUTCOMES

A number of studies examining the effect of individualized goal-setting with families for children with developmental problems or disabilities indicate significant relationships between supportive family decision making and collaborative goal-setting, and improved family and child functional outcomes (Dunst, Trivette, & Deal, 1988; Pomeranz, 1984; Cleary et al., 1991).

Starfield, Wray, Hess, Gross, Birk, and D'Lugoff (1981) studied agreement between people receiving ambulatory care through a health maintenance organization, and physicians and nurse practitioners. Ninety-four people began the study, and 41 received follow-up. The results of the study indicate that when the health care service provider and the client agreed on the focus of the problem, the client was more likely to indicate that the problem had been resolved at follow-up. The authors conclude that agreement between clients and health service providers is important to ensure that health problems are resolved.

Moxley-Haegert and Serbin (1983), in a randomized controlled trial, studied the effect of providing information and teaching to parents of infants with developmental delay. In this study, 39 parents were randomized to three groups: those who received education on child development in their home, general education in child management, and no education. Parents receiving developmental education participated more frequently in treatment programs and showed increased ability to provide information about their child's developmental skills to service providers. Children in the developmental education group also achieved significantly more skills on the motor domain of the Bayley Scales of Infant Development. Parker, Zahr, Cole, and Breck (1992) found similar outcomes for developmental intervention with pre-term infants.

In a cross-sectional study of 164, King, King, Rosenbaum, and Goffin (1997) used a structural equation modeling approach to investigate the factors that were associated with the emotional well-being of parents of children with disabilities. The results indicate that there is a significant causal relationship between the way in which care is provided and parent stress. Parents who perceived that the rehabilitation that their child was receiving was delivered in a more family-centred manner experienced less stress.

Rosenbaum, King, Law, King, and Evans (In press) have reviewed research evidence in pediatric studies to investigate the relationship between a family-centred approach to service delivery, and family and child outcomes. Studies were classified according to the level of evidence provided, ranging from Class I studies, which are randomized controlled trials, to Class II, which are cohort or before and after studies, Class III, which are cross-sectional or case-controlled studies, and Class IV, which includes descriptive or case studies. The results of this review indicate that there is strong evidence supporting the effect of family-centred approach to service on parent satisfaction. There is moderate to strong evidence suggesting that a family-centred approach to service can improve the outcomes of parents and functional outcomes for children.

Caro and Derevensky (1991) studied a family-focused intervention model with 16 families of infants with moderate to severe disabilities. Using a before and after study design, and both quantitative and qualitative methods, they evaluated outcomes after a 2-hour home visit per week for 5 months. Initially, an individualized family service plan was developed based on goals identified by each family. Intervention focused on providing information to parents about child development and how to facilitate their children's functional tasks, and facilitation of parent-infant interaction. Results indicated that children improved by an average of 4 months of age-adjusted performance on the Battell Developmental Inventory. Parent-infant interaction and parents' teaching skills also showed improvement. Qualitative analyses of parents' perspectives indicated that parents perceived that their children had important progress, and that they had developed new skills and supports for their role as parents of children with disabilities.

The effect of decision making by clients has been investigated by Kaplan (1991). Kaplan notes that making decisions about quality of life issues is often difficult for individuals because the effects of intervention are not always clear and involve making decisions about trade-offs. Occupational therapists don't always know all of the issues that influence clients' decisions. As Kaplan states, "their behaviour may be characterized by others as disrespectful of authority or as rebellious, but their choice, in fact, may reflect a careful balance between the health consequences and the social consequences of medicine use" (p. 72). While this quote relates to the choice of medicine by people with diabetes, it can also apply to choices that clients make during occupational therapy intervention. Kaplan reviews evidence showing that clients' perception of control has resulted in improved immune functioning and better health outcomes.

A study by Greenfield, Kaplan, and Ware (1985) indicates that people can be taught information about illnesses and that this information leads to improved outcome. In a randomized controlled trial, people with peptic ulcers were given a 20-minute intervention where they were taught to read their medical chart, and coached on how to question the doctor in negotiating decisions. After 6 weeks, the group that had received the intervention showed significantly improved satisfaction and fewer functional limitations. This study was replicated in people with diabetes (Greenfield, Kaplan, Ware, Yano, & Frank, 1988).

In a study of 415 clients of a health maintenance organization, Pitts, Schwankovsky, Thompson, Cruzen, Everett, and Freedman (1991) found that people receiving service wanted increased autonomy, particularly when choosing between equally effective interventions or when the effect of the intervention was not known. When the effect of the intervention is known or when increased technical knowledge is required to choose intervention, then people are more willing to let service providers make decisions about treatment. Kaplan (1991) states that "lack of information and control, not the possession of control, leads to irrational choice" (p. 86).

A recent randomized trial studied 651 clients older than 70 years of age who received usual medical care at a hospital or care in a unit focused on improving functional independence and using patient-centred care (Landefeld, Palmer, Kresevic, Fortinsky, & Kowal, 1995). In the unit focused on functional independence, the environment was structured to maintain and improve independence, specific protocols were used to improve functional assessment, and individualized programs were developed for intervention and discharge planning. Results of this study indicate that the group in the patient-centred independence unit were significantly more capable in functional performance and were less likely to be discharged to a long-term care institution.

Results of this review provide compelling evidence that the way in which services are delivered makes significant differences in adherence, client satisfaction, and functional outcome. The studies cited in this chapter demonstrate that delivering service in a client-centred manner, emphasizing client decision-making and client-service provider partnership, is more effective than services delivered in a traditional manner. The challenge for occupational therapists is to implement concepts of client-centred practice on a day-to-day basis.

Corring (1996) interviewed 17 individuals who had received occupational therapy services for mental illness. Through focus groups and a participatory action research approach, qualitative methods were used to gather information about the clients' perspective of client-centred concepts. The most important characteristics of client-centred practice perceived by these clients include being valued and treated with respect, perceiving a willingness of service providers to get to know the client and their concerns, a welcoming climate for service provision, taking the time to listen to clients, and developing an understanding between clients and service providers. Clients indicated that, although health service providers may espouse values of client-centred practice, moving these concepts into practice on a day-to-day basis is not always obvious to them as clients. Occupational therapists are not always seen as partners in changing environments that limit client-centred practice.

Consumers are demanding increased involvement and partnership in the delivery of occupational therapy services. Research evidence supports that a client-centred occupational therapy practice will lead to improved client satisfaction and outcomes. The implementation of client-centred occupational therapy on a day-to-day basis is challenging but worth the effort.

REFERENCES

Abramson, J. S. (1990). Enhancing patient participation: Clinical strategies in the discharge planning process. *Social Work and Health Care, 14*, 53-71.

Avis, M. (1994). Choice cuts: An exploratory study of patients' views about participation and decision-making in a day surgery unit. *International Journal of Nursing Studies, 31*, 289-298.

Ben-Sira, Z. (1976). The function of the professional's effective behaviour in client satisfaction: A revised approach to social interaction theory. *Journal of Health and Social Behaviour, 17*, 3.

Calnan, M., Katsouyiannopoulos, V., Ovcharov, V. K., Prokhorskas, R., Ramic, H., & Williams, S. (1994). Major determinants of consumer satisfaction with primary care in different health systems. *Family Practice, 11*(4), 468-478.

Canadian Association of Occupational Therapists. (1997). *Enabling occupation: An occupational therapy perspective.* Ottawa, ON: CAOT Publications ACE.

Caro, P., & Derevensky, J. L. (1991). Family-focused intervention model: Implementation and research findings. *Topics in Early Childhood Special Education, 11*(3), 66-80.

Cleary, P. D., Edgman-Levitan, S., Roberts, M., Moloney, T. W., McMullen, W., Walker, J. D., & Delbanco, T. L. (1991). Patients evaluate their hospital care: A national survey. *Health Affairs, 10*, 254-267.

Corring, D. J. (1996). *Client-centred care means I am a valued human being.* Masters of Science Thesis, University of Western Ontario, London, Ontario, Canada.

Doyle, B. J., & Ware, J. E. (1977). Physician conduct and other factors that affect consumer satisfaction with medical care. *Journal of Medical Education, 52*(10), 793-801.

Dunst, C. J., Trivette, C. M., Boyd, K., & Brookfield, J. (1994). Help-giving practices and the self-efficacy appraisals of parents. In C. J. Dunst, C. M. Trivette, K. Boyd, & J. Brookfield (Eds.). *Supporting and strengthening families: Methods, strategies and practices.* Vol. 1. Cambridge, MA: Brookline Books.

Dunst, C. J., Trivette, C. M., Deal, A. (1988). *Enabling and empowering families: Principles and guidelines for practice.* Cambridge, MA: Brookline Books.

Forchuck, C., & Roberts, J. (1993). How to critique qualitative research articles. *Canadian Journal of Nursing Research, 25*, 47-55.

Greenfield, S., Kaplan, S. H., & Ware, J. E. (1985). Expanding patient involvement in care: Effects on patient outcomes. *Annals of Internal Medicine, 102*, 520-528.

Greenfield, S., Kaplan, S. H., Ware, J. E., Yano, E. M., & Frank, H. J. (1988). Patients' participation in medical care: Effects on blood sugar control and quality of life in diabetes. *Journal of General Internal Medicine, 3*(5), 448-457.

Guyatt, G. H., Sackett, D. L., & Cook, G. J. (1993). The evidence-based medicine working group. User's guide to the medical literature. 1: How to use an article about therapy and prevention. *Journal of the American Medical Association, 270*, 2598-2601.

Henbest, R. J., & Fehrsen, G. S. (1992). Patient-centredness: Is it applicable outside the West? Its measurement and effect on outcomes. *Family Practice, 9*, 311-317.

Henbest, R. J., & Stewart, M. (1990). Patient-centredness in the consultation. 2: Does it really make a difference? *Family Practice, 7*(1), 28-33.

Huston, P. (1996). Cochrane Collaboration: Helping unravel tangled web woven by international research. *Canadian Medical Association Journal, 154*, 1389-1392.

Kaplan, R. (1991). Health-related quality of life and patient decision-making. *Journal of Social Issues, 47*, 69-90.

Kielhofner, G. (1995). *A model of human occupation: Theory and application* (2nd ed.). Baltimore: Williams and Wilkins.

King, G., King, S., Rosenbaum, P., & Goffin, R. (1997). Family-centred caregiving and well-being of parents of children with disabilities: Linking process with outcome. Manuscript in preparation.

King, G., King, S., & Rosenbaum, P. (1996). Interpersonal aspects of care-giving and client outcomes: A review of the literature. *Ambulatory Child Health, 2*, 151-160.

King, S., Rosenbaum, P., & King, G. (1996). Parents' perceptions of caregiving: Development and validation of a measure of processes. *Developmental Medicine and Child Neurology, 38*, 757-772.

Kirkhart, D. G. (1995). Shared care: Improving health care, reducing costs. *Nursing Management, 26*(6), 26-30.

Landefeld, C. S., Palmer, R. M., Kresevic, D. M., Fortinsky, R. H., & Kowal, J. (1995). A randomized trial of care and hospital medical unit especially designed to improve the functional outcomes of acutely ill older patients. *New England Journal of Medicine, 332*, 1338-1344.

Law, M. (1987). Criteria for the evaluation of measurement instruments. *Canadian Journal of Occupational Therapy, 54*, 121-127.

Law, M., Cooper, B., Strong, S., Stewart, D., Rigby, P., & Letts, L. (1996). The person-environment-occupation model: A transactive approach to occupational performance. *Canadian Journal of Occupational Therapy, 63*(1), 9-23.

Law, M., Cooper, B., Stewart, D., Letts, L., Rigby, P., & Strong, S. (1994). Person-environment relations. *Work, 4*, 228-238.

Lincoln, Y. S., & Guba, E. A. (1985). *Naturalistic enquiry.* Beverly Hills, CA: Sage Publications.

Marcenko, M. O., & Smith, L. K. (1992). The impact of a family-centred case management approach. *Social Work in Health Care, 17*(1), 87-100.

Moxley-Haegert, L., & Serbin, L. A. (1983). Developmental education for parents of delayed infants: Effects on parental motivation and children's development. *Child Development, 54*, 1324-1331.

Parker, S. J., Zahr, L. K., Cole, J. G., & Breck, M. L. (1992). Outcome after developmental intervention in the neo-natal intensive care unit for mothers of preterm infants with socioeconomic status. *Journal of Pediatrics, 120*, 780-785.

Patton, M. Q. (1990). *Qualitative evaluation and research methods* (2nd ed.). Newbury Park, CA: Sage Publications.

Pitts, J. S., Schwankovsky, L., Thompson, S. C., Cruzen, D. E., Everett, J., & Freedman, D. (1991, August). *Do people want to make medical decisions?* Paper presented at American Psychological Association meeting, San Francisco.

Pomeranz, B. P. (1984). Collaborative interviewing: A family-centred approach to pediatric care. *Health and Social Work, 9*, 66-73.

Rosenbaum, P., King, S., Law, M., King, G., & Evans, J. (In press). Family-centred service: A conceptual framework and research review. *Physical & Occupational Therapy in Pediatrics.*

Sackett, D. L. (1993). Rules of evidence and clinical recommendations. *Canadian Journal of Cardiology, 9*, 487-489.

Sackett, D. L., Haynes, R. B., Guyatt, G. H., & Tugwell, P. (1991). *Clinical epidemiology: A basic science for clinical medicine* (2nd ed.). Boston: Little, Brown and Company.

Starfield, B., Wray, C., Hess, K., Gross, R., Birk, P. S., & D'Lugoff, B. C. (1981). The influence of patient-practitioner agreement on outcome of care. *American Journal of Public Health, 71*, 127-132.

Stein, R. E. K., & Jessop, D. J. (1984). Does pediatric home care make a difference for children with chronic illness? Findings from the pediatric ambulatory care study. *Pediatrics, 73*, 845-853.

Stein, R. E. K., & Jones-Jessop, D. (1991). Long-term mental health effects of a pediatric home care program. *Pediatrics, 88*, 490-496.

Wasserman, R. C., Inui, T. S., Barriatua, R. D., Carter, W. B., & Lippincott, P. (1984). Pediatric clinicians' support for parents makes a difference: An outcome-based analysis of clinician-parent interaction. *Pediatrics, 74*(6), 1047-1053.

chapter

CLIENT-CENTRED PRACTICE IN A CHANGING HEALTH CARE SYSTEM

CAROLYN BAUM, PHD, OTR/C, FAOTA

A CHANGING HEALTH SYSTEM

Health care is expensive, and all professionals are being asked to reframe how care is delivered. Until now, the system has had an institutional orientation with the patient receiving services in a professionally driven model. The evolving model considers the person needing care a key part of the service, with the professional serving more as an educator and consultant. This is an enabling model rather than a prescriptive one, and requires occupational therapists to move beyond the medical model, which focuses on cure and management of the disease where the key relationship is between the patient and physician (Jesion & Rudin, 1983). The evolving model, called the social (community) model, focuses on the psychosocial as well as medical needs of individuals and encourages people to be as autonomous by providing opportunities for choice in decisions and activities (Smith & Eggleston, 1989). As community health initiatives, networks with independent living centers, schools, fitness and wellness programs, and vocational programs become recognized as means of maintaining the health of the community, occupational therapy will become even more integral to the system.

The team that has formed in the medical model has been limited to traditional medical rehabilitation professionals including physicians, occupational therapists, physical therapists, speech language pathologists, psychologists, and rehabilitation nurses. The community approach expands rehabilitation to include a whole new cadre of colleagues including people with disabilities, engineers, architects, personal assistants, independent living counselors, recreation and exercise personnel, city planners, law enforcement, and transportation specialists (Baum & Law, 1997).

The new paradigm (Figure 3-1) will emphasize the development of community partnerships where consumers and professionals will work together to develop strategies to manage health problems and prevent secondary disabling conditions that can compromise function.

There is another reason for these changes. The care needed by the one out of three citizens who has a chronic health or disabling condition is not necessarily a medical service. The services they require range from needing assistive devices like wheelchairs,

Old	New
The Model	
Medical model	Socio-political (community) model
Episodic care	Planned or managed health
The Focus	
Illness	Wellness
Acute care outcomes	Well-being, function, and life
Satisfaction	
Individual	Individual within the environment
Deficiency	Capability
Survival	Functional ability/quality of life
Professionally controlled	Personal responsibility
Flexible/choice	
Dependence	Interdependence/participation
Treatment	Treatment/prevention
The System	
Institution centred	Community centred
Single facility	Network
Competitive focus	Collaborative focus
Fragmented service	Coordinated service

Figure 3-1. Changing Health System Paradigm. Baum, C.M., & Law, M. (1997). Reprinted with permission of the American Occupational Therapy Association.

reachers, and bathtub railings, to having accessible housing and access to a barrier-free workplace and community (Institute for Health & Aging, 1996).

These changes challenge occupational therapists to extend their interventions beyond the clients' immediate impairments to focus on their long-term health needs by helping them develop behaviours to improve their health and well-being, and minimize long-term health care costs associated with dysfunction (Baum & Law, 1997). Thus, occupational therapists must view clients in the context of their lives and help them acquire the skills to handle not only the immediate issues that are influencing their health, but to learn strategies that will promote, protect, and improve their health over the long-term. This approach requires client- or family-centred services that extend from the agency or institution into the community.

The governments in Canada, the United States, and other countries have been working to improve the health and participation of their citizens through health promotion strategies (Health and Welfare Canada, 1986, 1987; US Department of Health and Human Services, 1990). Health is more than the absence of disease; it has evolved to include an emphasis on health promotion and disease prevention (World Health Organization, 1990). New initiatives are emerging with the goal of building healthy, supportive communities; reducing illness and disability; and improving the physical, social, and institutional environment (Premier's Council on Health, Well-Being and Social Justice, 1993; US Department of Health and Human Services, 1990). A number of the objectives associated with these agendas should call occupational therapists to action.

The stated goals include
- improving the functional independence of its citizens
- preventing the ill from becoming disabled
- encouraging physical activity
- reducing the number of people 65 and older who have difficulty performing two or more personal care activities
- reducing deaths caused by motor vehicle crashes
- reducing fall-related injuries
- increasing the proportion of providers of primary care who routinely evaluate people aged 65 and over for impairments of vision, hearing, cognition, and functional status

All of these objectives tap the knowledge and skills of occupational therapists. What is needed now are clear strategies for occupational therapists to use to make their contributions known and be recognized by primary care practitioners as a resource to support function and well-being. Client-centred practice is central to these strategies.

In the United States, the goal of prevention has not always been a feasible strategy for occupational therapists to implement because of limited mechanisms for payment. However, things are changing. The Joint Commission on Accreditation of Healthcare Organizations (JCAHO) is calling for health institutions to address the long-term health needs of those it serves (Joint Commission on the Accreditation of Healthcare Organizations, 1995). New community health guidelines implore health care institutions to assist in building healthier communities by helping patients and families foster environments conducive to recovery. This JCAHO initiative has two purposes: to promote health, and to decrease the long-term cost of care associated with chronic conditions. JCAHO is suggesting that a holistic approach is needed to respond to the diverse needs of an aging population, which it describes as having assessments and services that address physical, mental, emotional, and spiritual issues. This should stimulate community-based initiatives previously overlooked because occupational therapists in the United States were seen as a primary income source and were required to provide direct-billable services.

JCAHO also suggests that informal caregivers be included in educational opportunities offered by health care providers, and that they be given help in locating resources to use in providing care. JCAHO is asking health care systems to seek reimbursement for such care to avoid the risk of institutionalization. Additionally, it states that the health care system has a shared understanding of the roles, rights, and responsibilities of constituents. In other words, it recognizes that the client is a partner in the delivery of care. Occupational therapists must step forward to help people from other disciplines build these community-care initiatives.

A client-centred approach requires a different orientation, one that engages the assistance and support of a therapist to facilitate the client's problem solving and goal achievement (McColl, Gerein, & Valentine, 1997). This approach requires the therapist to move beyond a one-to-one approach into one of collaboration with individuals in the client's environment (family, teachers, independent-living specialists, employers, neighbours, and friends). A client-centred approach requires occupational therapy personnel to focus on the individual's needs and also to take an active role in building healthy communities (Baum & Law, 1997).

EMPLOYING A CLIENT-CENTRED APPROACH

Asking clients to be partners in their own care requires that the occupational therapist explore the extent to which clients feel that they can accomplish their objectives. Self-efficacy, or believing that a task or activity can be accomplished, allows one to feel effective and competent, which, in turn, contributes to improved occupational performance and well-being. Gage and Polatajko (1994) observed that perceived self-efficacy influences perseverance and well-being and that it can be modified through successful experiences that can be facilitated during occupational therapy.

Multiple factors contribute to illness and disability. Bandura (1977, 1978) has made a significant contribution to our understanding of the factors that influence health. His work in self-efficacy theory highlights the interacting determinants of behaviour, cognitive, and physiological and environmental influences to health. Self-efficacy theory postulates that the way people perceive their capabilities affects what they do, their level of motivation, their thought patterns, and their emotional reactions. Research has demonstrated that the effects of therapeutic interventions are partially mediated by a person's perceived self-efficacy (O'Leary, 1985).

Self-efficacy is at the core of client-centred practice. Occupational therapists need to frame their practice in models of care that focus on the clients' needs so that clients may gain motivation from their own perceptions and emotional efforts. Client-centred models are emerging. They will be discussed in the next section.

WHERE DOES CLIENT-CENTRED PRACTICE FIT IN THE LARGER ARENA OF REHABILITATION?

The individual is at the core of rehabilitation. Comprehensive client-centred models are beginning to emerge (Fougeyrollas, 1991; Figures 3-2 and 3-3) (NCMRR, 1993; Figures 3-4 and 3-5) to guide rehabilitation practice. These models support a client-centred practice and can be used by occupational therapists to organize assessments, design interventions, and plan services to meet the client's goals and needs. To implement a client-centred practice, emphasis must be placed at the level of the person-environment interaction. This interaction is addressed in the International Classification of Impairment, Disability, and Handicap model (ICIDH) at the disability, environmental factors, and life habit levels, and in the National Council for Medical Rehabilitation Research model (NCMRR) at the level of disabilities and societal limitations. A review of these models calls attention to the variables that must be addressed to impact the quality of life and well-being of the client and his or her family.

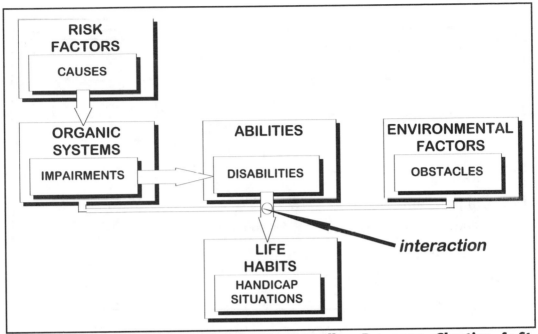

Figure 3-2. Modified ICIDH Model. ©Fougeyrollas, Bergeron, Cloutier, & St. Michel, 1991. Reprinted with kind permission from author, Patrick Fougeyrollas, PhD, President, Canadian Society for the ICIDH.

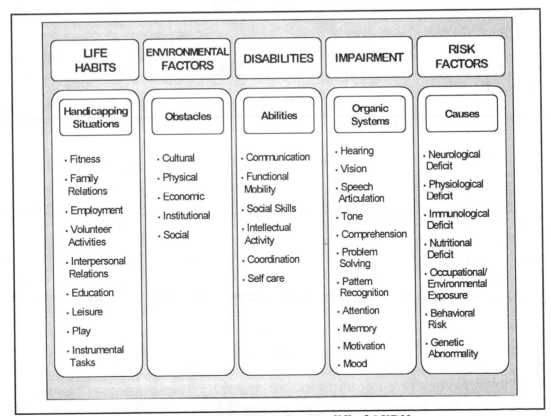

Figure 3-3. Measurement Model Using the Modified ICIDH.

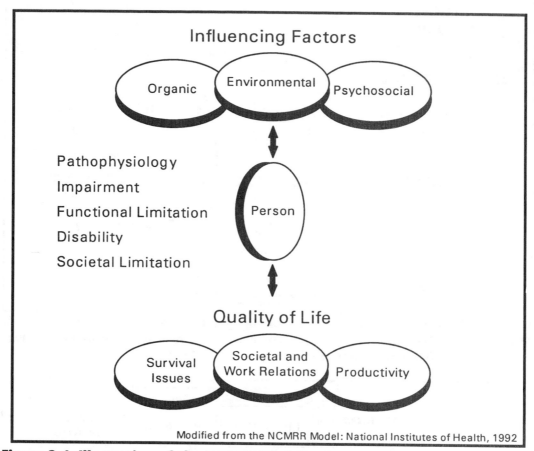

Figure 3-4. Illustration of the NCMRR Model.

OCCUPATION—THE CORE OF CLIENT-CENTRED PRACTICE

Occupational therapists view clients as individuals with unique characteristics and roles. People are usually characterized by what they do (Law, Cooper, Strong, Stewart, Rigby, & Letts, 1996). When their ability to do is compromised, their occupational performance is less satisfactory, and they can usually benefit from the services of an occupational therapist. The occupational therapist must come to understand the client's goals and skills in order to impact the client's occupational performance. This process evolves as a partnership.

During the past decade, a number of models of practice have emerged that address the person-environment occupational interaction (the contributing factors to occupational performance). Each of these models makes a unique contribution to our knowledge of occupation. It would be possible to assume that all occupational therapy models are client-centred. However, a model can only be described as client-centred when the

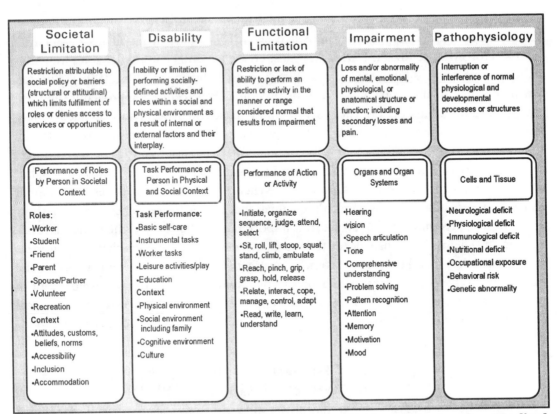

Societal Limitation	Disability	Functional Limitation	Impairment	Pathophysiology
Restriction attributable to social policy or barriers (structural or attitudinal) which limits fulfillment of roles or denies access to services or opportunities.	Inability or limitation in performing socially-defined activities and roles within a social and physical environment as a result of internal or external factors and their interplay.	Restriction or lack of ability to perform an action or activity in the manner or range considered normal that results from impairment	Loss and/or abnormality of mental, emotional, physiological, or anatomical structure or function; including secondary losses and pain.	Interruption or interference of normal physiological and developmental processes or structures
Performance of Roles by Person in Societal Context	Task Performance of Person in Physical and Social Context	Performance of Action or Activity	Organs and Organ Systems	Cells and Tissue
Roles: •Worker •Student •Friend •Parent •Spouse/Partner •Volunteer •Recreation **Context** •Attitudes, customs, beliefs, norms •Accessibility •Inclusion •Accommodation	**Task Performance:** •Basic self-care •Instrumental tasks •Worker tasks •Leisure activities/play •Education **Context** •Physical environment •Social environment including family •Cognitive environment •Culture	•Initiate, organize sequence, judge, attend, select •Sit, roll, lift, stoop, squat, stand, climb, ambulate •Reach, pinch, grip, grasp, hold, release •Relate, interact, cope, manage, control, adapt •Read, write, learn, understand	•Hearing •vision •Speech articulation •Tone •Comprehensive understanding •Problem solving •Pattern recognition •Attention •Memory •Motivation •Mood	•Neurological deficit •Physiological deficit •Immunological deficit •Nutritional deficit •Occupational exposure •Behavioral risk •Genetic abnormality

Figure 3-5. Measurement Model Built on the National Center for Medical Rehabilitation Research Scheme. Definitions modified by C. Baum, 1993, from work Initially developed by the Institute of Medicine and published in *Disability in America*, 1991, and reported in the *National Center for Medical Rehabilitation Research Plan*, NIH, 1993.

client seeks the assistance of a therapist, is actively encouraged to explain his or her problems, defines his or her needs, and experiences an environment of understanding, trust, and acceptance while pursuing his or her goals (Gerteis, Edgman-Levitan, Daley, & Delbanco, 1993). In the absence of an empowering environment where the clients direct the course of their care, long-term strategies to sustain the client and his or her family over the recovery or adaptation process are not possible.

In a client-centred approach, clients and therapists work together to define the nature of the occupational performance problems, the focus and need for intervention, and the preferred outcomes of therapy. Clients will participate at different levels, depending on their capabilities, but all are capable of making at least some choices about how they spend their daily lives (Baum & Law, 1997). The occupational therapist must have a fundamental respect for clients' values and visions and for their style of coping without being judgmental. Clients are encouraged to recognize and build on their strengths, using natural community supports as much as possible (Law, Baptiste, & Mills, 1995).

In order to be considered client-centred, occupational therapy models must consider the activities, tasks, and roles of the person (Christiansen & Baum, 1997); the organization of services to support the individual as an active participant in his or her care (Blank, Horowitz, & Matza, 1995); and must create a partnership that enables individuals to assume responsibility for their own care (Law, Baptiste, & Mills, 1995). The following occupational therapy models can be used in a client-centred approach if the therapist places the focus on the client's goals and the client's occupational needs (Law, Cooper, Strong, Stewart, Rigby, & Letts, 1997). Each of these models has the potential to evolve into a partnership between the occupational therapist and the client to address the client's goals. These models go far beyond the issues of performance components, but do not prohibit the therapist working with the client on strategies to address component issues that can influence the person's occupational performance. These models show great promise. As these models evolve, it is important that they extend their interventions beyond the client's immediate needs to help clients develop behaviours that avoid unnecessary secondary conditions and promote health that will support them in doing the things they want to do. Each needs further testing, and some require the development of more assessment tools; however, all are currently being studied and offer occupational therapy practitioners guidance in developing innovative and effective client-centred models of practice.

THE ECOLOGY OF HUMAN PERFORMANCE MODEL (DUNN, BROWN, & McGUIGAN, 1994)

This model focuses on context and how contextual factors such as physical, temporal, social, cultural, and/or phenomenology can impact the performance of the client. A client-centred approach is central to the identification of the tasks and activities that the person wants and needs to do. Instruments are being developed to support this model; these will ensure a strong orientation to the person-environment interaction and should make client-centredness very visible in the practice of the clinicians who subscribe to the model. This model helps the practitioner explore specific strategies to overcome the barriers that would limit the client's performance.

THE MODEL OF HUMAN OCCUPATION (KIELHOFNER & BURKE, 1980; KIELHOFNER, 1992, 1995)

This model evolved from Reilly's Model of Occupational Behavior (Reilly, 1966). The Model of Human Occupation (MOHO) focuses on occupational functioning and serves to guide practice in the organization or reorganization of occupational behaviour. Because it focuses on the client's routines and habits, the client's perspective and the client's motivation for activities must be determined. The person is viewed as a dynamic system influenced by the physical and social environment. MOHO has made significant contributions to occupational therapists' knowledge of clients' roles and how occupation is central to an individual's health. A number of interview instruments have been developed to support the model.

THE PERSON-ENVIRONMENT-OCCUPATION MODEL (LAW ET AL., 1996)

This transactive model considers the person, the occupation, and the environment in an interwoven relationship that views people in their everyday lives. The originators acknowledge that behaviour cannot be separated from contextual influences, temporal factors, and the physical and psychological characteristics of the person. They place their model in a developmental context, recognizing that environments, task demands, activities, and roles are constantly shifting. A person-environment-occupation intervention seeks to enable optimal occupational performance in occupations that are defined as important by the client. The authors of this model have explicitly stated the importance of focusing on the client's goals and sharing the process of the interaction to form a partnership that will assist the client in taking responsibility for his or her own rehabilitation. This model considers the Canadian Occupational Performance Measure (Law, Baptiste, Carswell, McColl, Polatajko, & Pollock, 1994) essential to its implementation; thus, the client's goals become the focus of the intervention.

THE PERSON-ENVIRONMENT-OCCUPATIONAL PERFORMANCE MODEL (CHRISTIANSEN & BAUM, 1991, 1997)

This model recognizes that the person's occupational performance cannot be separated from person-centred and contextual influences. It has operationalized the intrinsic factors (psychological, cognitive, physiological, and neuro-behavioural) and extrinsic or environmental factors (physical, cultural, social, and societal policies and attitudes) to understand the capacities of the individual to perform the activities, tasks, and roles that are important to the person. Additionally, the person's self-image, determined from competency, self-concept, and motivation, is considered in the overall plan for care that is driven by the client in a dynamic partnership with the clinician, and perhaps the family and others who are instrumental in the client's life. This approach requires that the practitioner determine the activities, tasks, and roles of the client to use as the central element in planning interventions and requires that the intervention engage the person in meaningful occupations as the process to support recovery or health maintenance.

OCCUPATIONAL ADAPTATION (SCHKADE & SCHULTZ, 1992)

This model has potential as a client-centred approach, as long as the activities chosen are client driven. The intervention uses a developmental framework that focuses on the importance that occupation plays in the life and maturation (of the development of competence) of the individual. This model encourages therapists to view a person holistically and to consider the client's internal processes and the environment. The model currently does not explicitly state that it focuses on the client's goals, but rather uses activities that are meaningful to the client to achieve the intervention goals. The model offers an important perspective that encourages occupational therapists to be creative and innovative in choosing activities that are meaningful to the client to achieve therapeutic goals. This model recognizes adaptations as central to the recovery process and occupation as the medium for therapy to produce that adaptation.

CONTEMPORARY TASK-ORIENTED APPROACH
(MATHIOWETZ & BASS HAUGEN, 1994)

This model integrates concepts from motor control, developmental, and motor learning theories to address the performance of functional tasks. A "top-down" approach to assessment and intervention considers the personal characteristics (cognitive, psychosocial, and sensorimotor) and the environmental context (physical, socioeconomic, and cultural) of the individual to determine the factors that limit occupational performance and then works to remove those limiting factors. This model shows great promise, and unlike earlier neuro-motor approaches, this model recognizes the critical nature of the client's goals for movement in the treatment approach.

CANADIAN MODEL OF OCCUPATIONAL PERFORMANCE
(CANADIAN ASSOCIATION OF OCCUPATIONAL THERAPISTS, 1997)

This model is a revised and updated version of the model in the Canadian Guidelines for Client-Centred Practice, which were originally published in 1981 (Department of National Health and Welfare & Canadian Association of Occupational Therapists, 1981). The model describes the relationship between people, their environments and occupations, and the process by which occupational therapists can enable clients to achieve optimal occupational performance. Spirituality, the innate essence of self, is a central construct in the model. This model is designed around a process to guide therapists in helping clients achieve satisfying levels of occupational performance.

Models of practice organized with a person, environment, and occupation focus have emerged in the past 15 years and, because they are conceptually compatible with the concept of community health and services that focus on health promotion and disease prevention, are gaining rapid acceptance in clinical practice. The scientists and practitioners contributing to these client-centred models are making an important contribution to the profession and also to the clients that the profession serves.

THE LIMITS OF TRADITIONAL MODELS OF PRACTICE

In the 1970s and 1980s, occupational therapists were trained to use biomechanical, acquisitional, sensorimotor, neurodevelopmental, and sensory integrative interventions that focused on the person with the goal of overcoming impairments that limited the potential for independent living. As the models supporting an occupation- and a client-centred focus orientation emerge, it may not be necessary to discard these approaches. However, the theoretical bases of these treatment approaches must be expanded to include social, cultural, physical, and societal factors to give context to the individual as he or she works to achieve his or her occupational roles. These models must also make explicit their focus of occupation in order to determine the importance of occupation to the client and to be considered as a client-centred approach.

The Rehabilitation Model has taken a huge step toward becoming a client-centred model by recognizing the critical role the environment plays in minimizing disability

(Brandt & Pope, 1997; Bickenbach, Ustun, & Chatterji). This places legitimate respon sibilities on occupational therapists to emerge in a leadership role by using environmental and assistive technologies to remove barriers that create unnecessary disabilities when people can't do what they want and need to do (occupation).

Other models may be able to make their way into a client-centred approach by making the role of occupation and the environment more explicit. Those approaches have been helpful in the past in conceptualizing an approach to treatment. They also fostered occupational definitions and identified measurement strategies to help the practitioner focus his or her treatment strategies. Unfortunately, it may have unnecessarily narrowed the focus of occupational therapy to the management of impairments (performance components) and encouraged therapists to make assumptions that reducing the impairment would result in increased function. In some cases this might be true, but this approach does not meet the criteria for being client-centred or even being considered rehabilitation unless how that impairment impacts everyday life is concurrently addressed in the intervention.

Now, as occupational therapists work from a client-centred community orientation, we are seeing the limits of narrowly focused practice models. A case in point:

Mrs. Jones has diabetes. She has been hospitalized and has received acute rehabilitation services and home health services. She was taught basic self-care and transfer techniques; she also received a bath bench, an extended shower head, a wheelchair, and a walker. Attention was focused on ensuring that she had the range of motion and skills to carry out her basic needs. Unfortunately, little attention was directed toward her functioning at home, particularly her loss of vision. Her husband is frail with a heart condition and needs skills to feel competent in his role. He reports that they are very isolated, and that his wife has become so dependent that he is required to perform even very simple personal tasks for her. He expresses worry that he may not be able to keep up the pace required to care for her much longer. So, rather than think of Mrs. Jones as the client, Mr. Jones must be seen not only as the environmental support of Mrs. Jones, but also as a client whose health may be compromised by the frustrations and tasks of his role.

The biomechanical and rehabilitative approaches did not go far enough because they focused on Mrs. Jones and her impairment and basic self-care function, not Mr. and Mrs. Jones as vulnerable older adults struggling to continue to live in their own home. Their issues go far beyond what traditional approaches support. A client-centred and occupation-based approach is needed. Such approaches will help them understand their options and how to integrate fitness, socialization, and meaningful occupations into their daily routines. The couple needs help that is available from community agencies like chore service, and assistance with shopping and transportation. The extended family also needs skills to develop competencies to help with some of the couple's needs.

In addition, there are a number of environmental strategies that can enhance the occupational performance of both Mr. and Mrs. Jones. The lighting in the home is too dim, and she needs some visual adaptations so she can read. Mr. Jones requires new strategies for transfers until Mrs. Jones gets stronger. Mrs. Jones also needs some of her clothes adapted so that she can dress more easily. Recently, she has remained in her robe all day and doesn't want neighbours to see her like that. Some additional assessments could help. The therapist suspects some depression and perhaps even early cognitive decline. It is also important to do an occupational history and determine the couple's interests and roles. These assessments can be done in the home and will be scheduled.

IMPLEMENTING CLIENT-CENTRED OCCUPATIONAL THERAPY SERVICES

In a client-centred program, the occupational therapist and the client bring important information to the partnership. When a therapeutic relationship is evolving, it is important for the relationship to be understood by both parties. It is just as important for clients to understand why the occupational therapist is involved in their care and what they can expect to achieve through occupational therapy, as it is for the therapist to understand the issues and needs of the client (Baum & Law, 1997). It is also important for clients to understand the scope of the therapist's knowledge. Additionally, the client's knowledge of his or her condition and experience with the problem must become clear for the relationship to progress. If a person has a cognitive limitation or is a child without the capacity for independent decision making, the parent or the person selected to be the guardian or caretaker must participate in treatment planning (Baum & Law, 1997) to ensure that the client's rights are protected.

The first phase of intervention should be designed to obtain information from the client about his or her perception of the problem, needs, and goals. An occupational performance history that includes information about the person, the environment, and the occupational factors that require occupational therapy intervention should be constructed. See Chapter 5 for discussion of a client-centred occupational therapy process.

The implementation of a client-centred approach requires us to use a top-down approach (Trombly, 1995; Mathiowetz & Bass Haugen, 1994) in which we determine what the clients perceive to be the important occupational performance issues that are causing them difficulty in carrying out their daily activities in work, self-maintenance, leisure, and rest (Baum & Law, 1997). Assessments are only part of the care; networks must be established with our colleagues in medicine and with the client, the family, and our colleagues in institutions and the community to ensure that the client makes the transition from the acute episode of care, through rehabilitation and community reintegration, to independent living (McColl, Gerein, & Valentine, 1997).

Occupational therapists have been socialized to make contributions to the rehabilitation process. The rehabilitation process has evolved to occur in institutions and be a time-limited process aimed at helping an impaired person reach an optimum level of function. This approach labels the recipient of service as a patient. It has also led the "patient" to understand that the therapist would be "fixing" the problem. The therapist expected patients and their families to comply with his or her recommendations and regularly attend if they expected to recover (McColl, Gerein, & Valentine, 1997).

To move from this traditional approach to a client-centred approach, we must shift from our focus on performance components to understand why problems occur and what might be done about them. The health system is requiring us to place a sharper focus on our unique contributions to health care. The unique contribution of occupational therapy is at the occupational performance level where the individual interacts with his or her environment to perform occupations and roles of choice.

The following are client-centred strategies that must be integrated into our current practice patterns to assume leadership in health systems that are changing to focus on the health of the people and the communities they serve.

- Adopt interventions to support the health and function of people in their communities. We have to ask ourselves how our interventions are improving the function and well-being of people, not just in basic self-care, but also in issues defined by them as important, like family, work, and leisure pursuits.

- Occupational therapy services should span from the institution to the community with specific services designed to maintain health and well-being for those with chronic disease and disability. We have to make sure there are places for people to engage in fitness and socialization activities. Productive pursuits must be central to our interventions, and services that help families acquire the skills to manage their loved ones' immediate and long-term needs must be central to our service delivery.

- Occupational therapists should form networks with independent-living centers, schools, fitness and wellness programs, and vocational rehabilitation. We must help our communities plan for the needs of people who will have more limitations in their ability to function. This offers opportunities for consultation on universal design and building accessible community centers and playgrounds, and requires occupational therapists to exercise their civic responsibilities in ensuring that communities are providing housing and services for a population with special needs.

- Occupational therapists should be seen as experts in applying effective intervention strategies that contribute to optimal occupational function, including self-sufficiency, social integration, improved health status, and employment of people with chronic disease and disability.

Our hospital systems are becoming community health systems. As they assume this role, the focus changes from one of providing acute medical care, to developing initiatives and promoting health and function that will prevent unnecessary hospitalizations and costs. This is prompted by the payment mechanism shift that eventually will lead to capitated rates where the health system will receive a fixed amount to provide all of the necessary health care for a population. This strategy requires that prevention become foremost in our approach. It also requires occupational therapists to adopt a strategy that integrates primary, secondary, and tertiary prevention into their practice and consultation patterns (Kniepmann, 1997).

If we apply a client-centred model from a community perspective, the occupational therapist would intervene much earlier and in different places in the delivery system. Figure 3-6 suggests some new opportunities for occupational therapists, all of which focus on the needs of people as they live their lives. Interventions that address these needs will require occupational therapists to explore payment in a broader context than insurance. We already have the experience of payment in schools; the next decade will bring expanded funds from industry as it seeks strategies to maintain productive workers. We will also create opportunities in the public health sector, as the strategies to help older adults remain in the community become more visible, and policies to support our children with interventions early in their development are developed.

We should take pride in our name "occupational therapist," a professional who practices in a client-centred context. As the health system reorganizes to serve a population with chronic disease and long-term health needs, we have a rich history as a profession organized around the principles that are now being demanded for the health professionals of the future. The Pew commission (Shugars, O'Neil, & Bader, 1991) has described the health practitioner of the future as one who:

- Cares for the community's health. They believe that practitioners should have a broad understanding of the environmental factors, socio-economic conditions, and behaviours that influence health and should be able to work with others in the community to integrate a range of services that promote, protect, and improve the health of the public.
- Emphasizes primary care. They are challenging practitioners to function in new health care settings and interdisciplinary teams to meet the primary health care needs of the public.
- Participates in coordinated care. They are challenging practitioners to work effectively as team members in programs that emphasize high-quality, cost-effective integrated services.
- Practices prevention. The emphasis should expand to incorporate primary, secondary, and tertiary preventive strategies for all people.
- Involves patients and families in the decision-making process. They challenge practitioners to actively engage patients and their families in decisions regarding their personal health care, and in evaluating its quality and acceptability.
- Promotes healthy lifestyle. Practitioners should help individuals, families, and communities maintain and promote healthy behaviour.

Consumer	Needs
Industry	Productive workers
Social Security Administration	Functional capacities evaluations
Hospital/community health system	Prevention of secondary conditions
Schools	Children with the capacity to learn
City and county government	Capacity for community living
Architecture and engineering firms	Assistive environments and technology
Penal institution	Opportunities for work and recovery
Public information	Health information
Universities	Research and knowledge dissemination
Adult learning centers	Knowledgeable consumers
Retirement communities	Independence in the least restrictive environment
Day care facilities (child and adult)	Avoid excess disability

Figure 3-6. Opportunities for Occupational Therapy Intervention.

These behaviours have always been central to occupational therapy practice and can best be implemented in a client-centred approach. The challenge of the Pew Commission offers occupational therapists the opportunity to practice within the framework of their core values and make the contribution of occupation to health visible.

1. Engagement in occupation is valuable because it provides opportunities for individuals to influence their well-being by gaining fulfillment in living.

2. Through the experience of occupation (or doing), the individual is able to achieve mastery and competence by learning skills and strategies necessary for coping with problems and adapting to limitations.

3. As competence is gained and autonomy can be expressed, independence is achieved.

4. Autonomy implies choice and control over environmental circumstances. Thus, opportunities for exerting self-determination should be reflected in intervention strategies.

5. Choice and control extend to decisions about intervention, thus identifying occupational therapy as a collaborative process between the therapist and recipient of care. In this collaboration, the person's values are respected.

6. Because of its focus on life performance, occupational therapy is neither somatic, nor psychological, but concerned with the unity of body and mind in doing. (Baum & Christiansen, 1997).

BUILDING THE FUTURE

The health care system is offering occupational therapists a challenge to improve the health and function of the population. We can look at this challenge as a threat to our practice today, or we can see it as an opportunity to implement what the founders of occupational therapy envisioned—creating opportunities for people to lead independent and healthful lives.

Occupational therapy practice must focus on occupational performance, assisting our clients in becoming actively engaged in their life activities. This requires us to build a client-centred and family-centred practice and extend our services from the agency or institution into the community. We must work collaboratively with individuals in the client's environment (teachers, independent-living specialists, employers, neighbours, friends) to assist the client with the modifications that will remove barriers that would put him or her at a social disadvantage. This requires all occupational therapy personnel to take an active role in their communities. As Mary Reilly said in her Eleanor Clarke Slagel lecture: The future is very bright for a profession that "... has as its unique concern, the nurturing of the spirit ... for action" (1962, p. 92).

REFERENCES

Bandura, A. (1977). *Social learning theory*. Englewood Cliffs, NJ: Prentice-Hall.

Bandura, A. (1978). The self-system in reciprocal determinism. *American Psychologist, 33*, 344-359.

Baum & Christiansen (1997). The occupational therapy context: Philosophy-principles-practice. In C. Christiansen & C. Baum, *Occupational therapy: Overcoming human performance deficits*. Thorofare, NJ: SLACK Incorporated, pp. 4-43.

Baum, C. M., & Law, M. (1997). Occupational therapy practice: Focusing on occupational performance. *American Journal of Occupational Therapy, 51*(4), 277-288.

Bickenbach, J. E., Ustun, T. B., & Chatterji, S. (submitted). The social model of disablement, universalism and the ICIDH. *Disability and Society*.

Blank, A.E., Horowitz, S., & Matza, D. (1995). Quality with a human face? The Samuels Planetree Model hospital unit. *Journal of Quality Improvement, 21*, 289-299.

Brandt, E. N., & Pope, A. M. (Eds.) (1997). *Enabling America: Assessing the role of rehabilitation science and engineering*. Washington, DC: National Academy Press.

Canadian Association of Occupational Therapists. (1997). *Enabling occupation: an occupational therapy perspective*. Ottawa, ON: CAOT Publications ACE.

Christiansen, C., & Baum, C. (1991). *Occupational therapy: Overcoming human performance deficits*. Thorofare, NJ: SLACK Incorporated, pp. 4-43.

Department of National Health and Welfare and Canadian Association of Occupational Therapists (1981). *Guidelines for the client-centred practice of occupational therapy*. Ottawa, ON: Department of National Health and Welfare.

Dunn, W., Brown, C., & McGuigan, A. (1994). Ecology of human performance: A framework for considering the effect of context. *American Journal of Occupational Therapy, 48*(7), 595-607.

Fougeyrollas, P. (1991). Applications of the concept of handicap and its nomenclature. *ICIDH and Environmental Factors International Network, 6*(3), 24-48.

Gage, M., & Polatajko, H. (1994). Enhancing occupational performance through an understanding of perceived self-efficacy. *American Journal of Occupational Therapy, 48*(5), 452-462.

Gerteis, M., Edgman-Levitan, S., Daley, J., & Delbanco, T.L. (1993). *Through the Patient's Eyes: Understanding and promoting patient-centred care*. San Francisco: Jossey-Bass Publishers.

Health and Welfare Canada (1986). *Achieving health for all: a framework for health promotion*. Ottawa, ON: Government of Canada.

Health and Welfare Canada (1987). *Active health report*. Ottawa, ON: Government of Canada.

Jesion, M., & Rudin, S. Evaluation of the social model of long term care. *Health Management Forum, Summer*, 1983, 64-80.

Joint Commission on the Accreditation of Healthcare Organizations (1995). *Assessing and improving community health care delivery*. Oakbrooke Terrace, IL: Author.

Kielhofner, G. (1992). *Conceptual foundations of occupational therapy*. Philadelphia: F. A. Davis.

Kielhofner, G. (1995). *A model of human occupation: Theory and application* (2nd ed.). Baltimore: Williams & Wilkins.

Kielhofner, G., & Burke, J. (1980). A model of human occupation, part one: Conceptual framework and content. *American Journal of Occupational Therapy, 34,* 572-581.

Kniepmann, K. (1997). Prevention of disability and maintenance of health. In C. Christiansen & C. Baum (Eds.). *Occupational therapy: Enabling function and well-being* (2nd ed.) Thorofare, NJ: SLACK Incorporated.

Law, M., Baptiste, S., Carswell, A., McColl, M., Polatajko, H., & Pollock, N. (1994). *Canadian occupational performance measure* (2nd ed.). Toronto, ON: CAOT Publication.

Law, M., Baptiste, S., & Mills, J. (1995). Client-centred practice: What does it mean and does it make a difference? *Canadian Journal of Occupational Therapy, 62,* 250-257.

Law, M., Cooper, B. A., Strong, S., Stewart, D., Rigby, P., & Letts, L. (1996). The person-environment-occupation model: A transactive approach to occupational performance. *Canadian Journal of Occupational Therapy, 63,* 9-23.

Law, M., Cooper, B. A., Strong, S., Stewart, D., Rigby, P., & Letts, L. (1997). Theoretical context for the practice of occupational therapy. In C. Christiansen & C. Baum (Eds.), *Occupational therapy: Enabling function and well-being* (2nd ed.). Thorofare, NJ: SLACK Incorporated.

Mathiowetz, V., & Bass Haugen, J. (1994). Motor behavior research: Implications for therapeutic approaches to central nervous system dysfunction. *American Journal of Occupational Therapy, 48,* 733-745.

McColl, M. A, Gerein, N., & Valentine, F. (1997). Meeting the challenges of disability. Models for enabling function and well-being. In C. Christiansen & C. Baum (Eds.) *Occupational therapy: Enabling function and well-being* (2nd ed.). Thorofare, NJ: SLACK Incorporated.

NCMRR (1993). *Research plan for the National Center for Medical Rehabilitation Research.* (NIH Publication No. 93-3509). National Institutes of Health, Washington, DC: US Government Printing Office.

O'Leary, A. (1985). Self efficacy and health. *Behavioral Research and Therapy, 23*(4), 437-451.

Premier's Council on Health, Well-Being and Social Justice (1993). *Our environment, our health.* Toronto, ON: Province of Ontario.

Reilly, M. (1962). Occupational therapy can be one of the great ideas of 20th century medicine. *The American Journal of Occupational Therapy, 16,* 92.

Reilly, M. (1966). The challenge of the future to an occupational therapist. *The American Journal of Occupational Therapy, 20,* 221-225.

Institute for Health & Aging (1996). E. Freudenheim (Ed.). *Chronic care in America: A 21st century challenge.* Princeton, NJ: The Robert Wood Johnson Foundation.

Schkade, J. K., & Schultz, S. (1992). Occupational adaptation: Toward a holistic approach to contemporary practice. Part I. *American Journal of Occupational Therapy, 46,* 829-837.

Shugars, D. A., O'Neil, E.H., Bader, J.D. (Eds.) (1991). *Healthy America: Practitioners for 2005, an agenda for action for U.S. health professional schools.* Durham, NC: The Pew Health Professions Commission.

Smith, V., & Eggleston, R. (1989). Long-term care The medical versus the social model. *Public Welfare, Summer,* 26-29.

Trombly, C. A. (1995).Occupation: Purposefulness and meaningfulness and therapeutic mechanisms. *American Journal of Occupational Therapy, 49,* 960-972.

US Department of Health and Human Services. Public Health Services (1990). *Healthy People 2000—National Health Promotion and Disease Prevention Objectives.* DHHS Publication No.(PHS) 91-50212. Washington, DC: US Government Printing Office.

World Health Organization (WHO) (1990). *Healthy cities—Action strategies for health promotion, first project brochure.* Copenhagen: Author.

chapter

4

CLIENT-CENTRED OCCUPATIONAL THERAPY: THE CANADIAN EXPERIENCE

ELIZABETH TOWNSEND, PhD, OT(C)

Canadian occupational therapists will close the 20th century with a 20-year history of developing guidelines for client-centred occupational therapy practice. Client-centred practice in Canada has emerged in a context marked by long-standing collaboration amongst occupational therapists and clients, and between the Canadian Association of Occupational Therapists (CAOT), the Canadian government, and other organizations. Like occupational therapists everywhere, Canadians know that practice is most meaningful and useful when it focuses on client goals and involves clients as participants who are collaborators in the process. Reflecting on the writings of Carl Rogers and others, Canadian occupational therapists recognize that occupational therapy, at its best, is essentially client-centred. A 1990 article, *Developing Guidelines for Client-Centred Occupational Therapy Practice,* outlined the historical development of the first three volumes of Canadian guidelines on client-centred practice (Townsend, Brintnell, & Staisey, 1990). This chapter is a history of the national collaboration that has made client-centred practice an important part of Canadian occupational therapy. Its four sections summarize historical highlights in shifting from quality assurance in the 1960s and 1970s to outcome measurement in the 1980s; five processes facilitating the development of a Canadian occupational therapy perspective for the 1990s and beyond; four decades of collaboration; and two core notions emerging in client-centred practice. Eight scenarios are interspersed to illustrate ways of making client-centred practice a reality. This historical chapter is included so that occupational therapists around the world may learn from the Canadian experience.

FROM QUALITY ASSURANCE TO OUTCOME MEASUREMENT: THE 1960s TO THE 1980s

ACTIVITIES PROMPTING INTEREST IN CLIENT-CENTRED PRACTICE

In Canada, an orientation to client-centred practice grew out of government and professional concerns to evaluate health services and to make services more accountable through quality assessment and quality assurance. Four activities by CAOT, from 1966 to 1979, prompted the formation of task forces, which produced Canada's 1980s guidelines for client-centred practice in occupational therapy (Department of National Health and Welfare and Canadian Association of Occupational Therapists, 1983). The first activity was to develop a national workload measurement system (Management Information Systems Group, 1993). The second related activity was CAOT's development, beginning in 1973, of standards for occupational therapy services. Oriented for use in hospital accreditation, initial standards outlined a quality structure, but not a quality process or outcomes for occupational therapy (Canadian Council on Hospital Accreditation, 1977). Of note, the 1990s standards for occupational therapy in rehabilitation services now advocate a client-centred approach (Canadian Council for Health Services Accreditation, 1995). A third activity to increase occupational therapy accountability began in 1977 (Bridle, 1977), when CAOT sponsored the development of the Occupational Therapist-Occupational Profile, which was used well into the 1980s in Canadian academic and field-work education (Bridle, 1981). Establishing task forces to develop practice guidelines was CAOT's fourth activity. The chairperson of CAOT's Council on Practice prompted CAOT officials to apply for funding from the Clinical Guidelines Program in the Institutional and Professional Services Branch of the Health Services Directorate in the Department of National Health and Welfare (DNHW).

THREE VOLUMES OF NATIONAL GUIDELINES AND RELATED PROJECTS

Starting in December 1979, a task force, sponsored jointly by the CAOT and Canada's DNHW, began to develop national guidelines for occupational therapy practice. Its 11 members brought academic, hospital, community, government, and professional perspectives on occupational therapy and a history of active involvement in the work of this profession (Department of National Health and Welfare and Canadian Association of Occupational Therapists, 1983). Of interest, the Terms of Reference that were developed at the first meeting were not oriented to client-centred practice. Nevertheless, after 10 meetings over more than 3 years, and an extensive review of occupational therapy, quality assurance, programme evaluation, accreditation standards, health promotion, disability, sociology, psychology, professionalism, and related literature from the 1960s to the mid-1980s, a document, *Guidelines for the Client-Centred Practice of Occupational Therapy* was submitted (Department of National Health and Welfare and Canadian Association of Occupational Therapists, 1983). These guidelines provided

> "... a conceptual framework for occupational therapy, Canada-wide general guidelines for practice, and specific guidelines for assessment and program planning. These consensus guidelines which are unanimously supported by the Task Force represent the completion of Stage I of the project. The Task Force recommends that Stage II be initiated to develop detailed intervention guidelines." (Department of National Health and Welfare and Canadian Association of Occupational Therapists, 1983, p. xi)

Reviewed in these guidelines were quality-care measures and the task force's reasons for starting with process, not outcome or structure, as defined by Donabedian (1966). With guidelines for the structure of hospital-based occupational therapy services already incorporated in hospital accreditation, process guidelines were viewed as a necessary "first step in identifying and describing the sequential interaction of events of the client with the occupational therapist" (Department of National Health and Welfare and Canadian Association of Occupational Therapists, 1983, p. 4). The guidelines were client-centred, not profession-centred, because they recognized individuals' responsibility for their own health and because they described a seven-stage process for working with clients, from referral to evaluation. Occupational therapists' wide ranging skills, ethics, therapeutic relationship, multidisciplinary team work, and creativity were described as fundamental to each stage of the process even though they were not, in themselves, indicators of quality or accountability. Moreover, these were consensus guidelines that presented a vision of "reasonable as opposed to optimal or minimal" practice (Department of National Health and Welfare and Canadian Association of Occupational Therapists, 1983, p. 2). Known also as generic guidelines, they presented a general process that could be applied in the many diverse types of occupational therapy practice. They were guidelines, not standards, because Canadian provinces define and monitor standards through provincial organizations, such as those that regulate occupational therapy practice. The federal role was to provide guidelines that offer "outlines, suggestions, or benchmarks which may be modified and developed into standards" (Department of National Health and Welfare and Canadian Association of Occupational Therapists, 1983, p. 2). Consensus guidelines were preferred over standards that are out of date almost before they are printed, need constant revision, and are costly to enforce. They were developed as conceptual guidelines with a conceptual framework to guide processes that differ with each client, environment, and other factors. In summary, their purpose was to foster cohesiveness, consistency, and high standards across diverse areas of practice; form the basis of quality assurance and programme evaluation in occupational therapy across Canada; articulate a generic, conceptual framework for clinical, administrative, and educational programme planning and research; support a nationally consistent orientation to student occupational therapists; and provide an important resource for public relations to inform those in government, other professions, and the community about occupational therapy.

Client-centred practice was not explicitly defined; instead, five theoretical and philosophical concepts of client-centred practice were presented (Table 4-1): worth of the individual, holistic view of man [sic], occupational performance model, therapeutic use of activity, and developmental perspective. In highlighting the worth of the individual, occupational therapists were reminded that all individuals have a capacity to interpret, mediate, and act in reaching their potential; they were also reminded that a client-centred occupational therapist takes a holistic view of man [sic], as displayed on early Canadian uniforms with a triangular arm badge depicting the interaction of mind, body, and spirit (Trent, 1919). Canada's first Occupational Performance Model (OPM) supported the view of an active, participating client by graphically showing an individual interacting in the environment in three areas of occupation, namely self-care, productivity, and leisure. The OPM drew particularly on the work of Reed and Sanderson (1980) to provide a sim-

Table 4-1
1983 Conceptual Foundations of Occupational Therapy's Client-Centred Practice

Concept	Client-Centred Practice
Worth of the Individual	Clients are active participants
Holistic View of [Man] the Individual	Individuals are integrated in body-mind-spirit
Occupational Performance Model	Focus on occupational performance, not body parts
Therapeutic Use of Activity	Health promoted through engagement in activity
Developmental Perspective	Change through developmental processes
Process of Practice	Client participates in each stage

ple, clear graphic that recognized occupational performance as a central focus and incorporated the environment as well as individual performance in occupational therapy's domain of practice. Concepts about the therapeutic use of activity and a developmental perspective were included to emphasize that occupational therapists involve clients in *activity* (today we would refer to *occupation*) with recognition that individuals progress through developmental stages. A systems view of practice was offered as a way of showing how feedback prompts adaptation in individuals, their environment, their areas of occupational performance, and the processes they are engaged in with an occupational therapist. An occupational therapy process that incorporated these five concepts of client-centred practice was defined in seven stages: referral, assessment, programme planning, intervention, discharge, follow-up, and evaluation.

Between 1984 and 1986, a second task force produced *Intervention Guidelines for the Client- Centred Practice of Occupational Therapy* (Department of National Health and Welfare and Canadian Association of Occupational Therapists, 1986). It is important to note that these guidelines deliberately referred to intervention, not treatment. Canadian occupational therapists were expanding rapidly outside medical contexts; and client-centred practice involves collaboration with, versus doing for, people as is implied in treatment. To illustrate, enabling a frail, elderly woman to organize neighbourhood help, discover meaningful occupations, and physically adapt her home for living with mobility restrictions is not treatment, but rather intervention, or the implementation of plans developed with her.

Table 4-2
1986 Conceptual Foundations for Client-Centred Intervention in Occupational Therapy

---

FUNDAMENTAL ELEMENTS

Spirituality

Motivation

Therapeutic Relationship

Teaching Learning Process

Ethics

ORIENTING PRINCIPLES

Professionalization

Team Concept

Adaptation: Prevent Dysfunction, and Develop, Restore, Maintain Function

CONCEPTS OF CLIENT-CENTRED PRACTICE

Worth of the Individual

Holistic View of the Individual

Occupational Performance Model

Therapeutic Use of Activity

Developmental Perspective

Process of Practice

The second guidelines document expanded understanding of client-centred practice by describing three orienting principles and five fundamental elements of client-centred intervention (Table 4-2) flowing from the fundamental concepts of client-centred practice introduced in *Guidelines for the Client-Centred Practice of Occupational Therapy* (Department of National Health and Welfare and Canadian Association of Occupational Therapists, 1983). The orienting principles were professionalization, team approach, and adaptation. The orientation of occupational therapy, as seen in 1986, was to enable adaptation in individuals and environments so that individuals can develop, restore, or maintain function, or prevent dysfunction.

Five fundamental elements for client-centred intervention in occupational therapy were described as: *spirituality, motivation, therapeutic relationship, teaching learning process,* and *ethics.* Spirituality was highlighted to underscore the importance of attending to meaning in clients' lives. Of note, spiritual malaise or anomie was differentiated from the psychological construct of motivation. Individuals were recognized as having a spirit, as well as a body and a mind. Motivation, on the other hand, was recognized as a psychological process related to self-concept, confidence, and sense of control in making decisions. The guidelines suggested that occupational therapists attend to spirituality by asking clients what is meaningful and by orienting intervention and other stages of the process to that meaning. Motivation was highlighted as something that "challenges the passive 'patient' roles as no longer adaptive" (Department of National Health and Welfare and Canadian Association of Occupational Therapists, 1986, p. 15). The therapeutic relationship was described as a process that conveys concern for the client and establishes collaborative communication in which there is trust in clients' as well as occupational therapists' knowledge. Throughout the initiation, working phase, and termination of the therapeutic relationship, occupational therapists and clients were said to engage in a mutual process of teaching and learning: clients learn from occupational therapy expertise, but occupational therapists also learn from clients' experiences and self-knowledge. Rather than treating people, this collaborative process involves education and learning, with risk taking, problem solving, decision making, skill acquisition, and other approaches for learning to adjust through processes of change. Ethics were included as an element of intervention because client-centred practice attends to clients' values and beliefs in what *ought* to be done. The ethical element is central to client-centred practice given that clients and occupational therapists may hold differing values and beliefs about goals and priorities. Highlighted was the importance of occupational therapists upholding their professional responsibilities to both serve clients' needs while also adhering to the profession's code of ethics to ensure that potential harm to clients is minimized.

A third guidelines document, *Toward Outcome Measures in Occupational Therapy,* was released in 1987. In these guidelines, a review of outcome measures in self-care, productivity, and leisure was summarized; issues in measuring efficiency, effectiveness, and cost-benefit were highlighted; results of a national survey were presented, indicating that self-care and leisure were addressed more frequently even though household management and productivity are viewed as important outcomes; and principles for developing an assessment tool of occupational performance that would be compatible with client-centred practice were listed. Like previous guidelines, these were not "how to" guidelines; rather they offered a state-of-the-art overview of outcome measurement pertinent to occupational therapy in the late 1980s. They indicated that self-care, productivity, and leisure are the primary outcomes of occupational therapy, while physical, mental, and socio-cultural performance components are secondary outcomes, i.e., a means to the real outcomes of occupational therapy. This view of occupational therapy has since been depicted as highly compatible with the World Health Organization's International Classification of Impairments, Disabilities, and Handicaps (Townsend, Ryan, & Law, 1990).

Recommendations for the client-centred measurement of occupational performance outcomes were then incorporated in a new assessment tool, the Canadian Occupational Performance Measure (COPM) (Law, Baptiste, Carswell, McColl, Polatajko, & Pollock, 1994; Law, Baptiste, McColl, Opzoomer, Polatajko, & Pollock, 1990). Being client-centred, the COPM does not measure occupational therapy outcomes; rather it focuses on occupational performance outcomes in an individual's self-care, productivity, and leisure as defined and rated by a client in terms of importance, performance, and satisfaction.

As the 1990s began, Canadian occupational therapists had three guidelines documents and the COPM to promote quality, client-centred practice (Townsend, Brintnell, & Staisey, 1990). Local, provincial, and national uses are illustrated in scenarios #1, #2, and #3.

Scenario #1: Performance Appraisal of Client-Centred Practice

An occupational therapist is participating with a supervisor in performance appraisal. Observation indicates that the occupational therapist shows enthusiasm with clients and spends a lot of time preparing projects so that clients experience success in seeing a finished product. Yet, there is almost no record keeping; assessment, planning, follow-up, and evaluation are rarely done; and the occupational therapist generally turns down opportunities for continuing professional education, claiming to be too busy. With the three sets of guidelines and the COPM readily at hand, the supervisor reminds the occupational therapist that quality occupational therapy practice focuses on restoring, developing, or maintaining function, or preventing dysfunction in occupational performance as depicted in the Occupational Performance Model. *Quality* means that clients are satisfied with changes in performance or satisfaction in the self-care, productivity, or leisure areas that they have defined as being most important. Moreover, quality is demonstrated by following and documenting the seven-stage process of practice with notes that refer to the therapeutic use of activity, spirituality, motivation, and the therapeutic relationship. The occupational therapist is advised to become familiar with these tools, to keep clear records that describe how a quality process and relevant outcomes are addressed, and to take time for continuing professional education rather than preparing projects that may not be related to clients' needs.

Scenario #2: Educating Client-Centred Practitioners

An occupational therapy educational program is revising its curriculum. Faculty and fieldwork preceptors agree that courses that focus on specific medical diagnoses do not prepare students to apply occupational therapy theories and principles in the wide ranging situations that practitioners encounter. The curriculum planning group remembers that Canadian occupational therapists have generic, conceptual guidelines for client-centred practice, which focus on occupational performance. Committee members say that it makes sense to educate students in the conceptual framework, orienting principles, and fundamental elements of occupational therapy, so that they can work anywhere yet stay focused on their contribution to the team as occupational therapists. The curriculum planning group proposes that students learn how occupational performance develops over the lifespan, how change can be facilitated in environments as well as individuals, and how meaningful outcomes emerge when spirituality and motivation are addressed. In both the classroom and fieldwork education, students are encouraged to develop collaborative relationships and to openly discuss ethical conflicts between what clients want to do, and what occupational therapists and other professionals think is appropriate.

Scenario #3: Embedding Client-Centred Practice in National and Provincial Documents

CAOT decided in the mid-1980s to incorporate client-centred guidelines in national policies and the National Certification Examination. A national Client-Centred Practice Committee was established to promote use of the guidelines and to update them as needed. The first National Certification Examination Committee required examination scenarios and multiple choice answers that refer to occupational performance and clients (not patients). The *Canadian Journal of Occupational Therapy* now encourages submissions that examine concepts, processes, and outcomes of occupational performance. CAOT position papers on areas of specialization in occupational therapy are being developed with reference to the Occupational Performance Model, highlighting client participation in the occupational therapy process, regardless of the frames of reference or intervention methods used. CAOT's fieldwork and academic accreditation standards have included the guidelines as key undergraduate reference materials. In addition, CAOT has arranged for guidelines to be distributed to key organizations and individuals for international reviews, presentations, or other uses. Increasingly, CAOT is incorporating concepts, principles, and elements of client-centred practice in its policies, funding priorities, conference themes, publication priorities, and promotions. Provincial regulatory and professional bodies are gradually embedding client-centred practice in their documents.

DEVELOPING A CANADIAN OCCUPATIONAL THERAPY PERSPECTIVE: THE 1990s AND BEYOND

In the 1990s, a vision of occupational therapy concepts, discourse, and strategies for client-centred practice was promoted by CAOT through five, interrelated initiatives presented in Table 4-3 as consolidating, clarifying, concentrating, classifying, and creating.

CONSOLIDATING

A 1991 edition, *Occupational Therapy Guidelines for Client-Centred Practice* (Canadian Association of Occupational Therapists, 1991), consolidated the 1983 (Department of National Health and Welfare and Canadian Association of Occupational Therapists, 1983), 1986 (Department of National Health and Welfare and Canadian Association of Occupational Therapists, 1986), and 1987 (Department of National Health and Welfare and Canadian Association of Occupational Therapists, 1987) guidelines in gender neutral language, removing duplicate references, and updating glossary definitions. The pref-

Table 4-3
The 1990s: Five Interrelated Initiatives

Consolidating	**Consolidating the original guidelines** Canadian Association of Occupational Therapists. *Occupational Therapy Guidelines for Client-Centred Practice*. Toronto, ON: Author; 1991.
Clarifying	**Clarifying uses and usefulness of the original guidelines** Blain, J. & Townsend, E. Occupational therapy guidelines for client-centred practice: Impact study findings. *Canadian Journal of Occupational Therapy*. 1993; 60:271-285.
Concentrating	**Concentrating on guidelines for mental health practice** Health Canada and Canadian Association of Occupational Therapists. *Occupational Therapy Guidelines for Client-Centred Mental Health Practice*. Ottawa, ON: Minister of Supply and Services; 1993.
Classifying	**Classifying areas of professional competence** Canadian Association of Occupational Therapists. Profile of Occupational Therapy practice in Canada. *Canadian Journal of Occupational Therapy*. 1996; 63:79-113.
Creating	**Creating new guidelines** Canadian Association of Occupational Therapists. *Enabling Occupation: A Canadian Occupational Therapy Perspective*. Ottawa, ON: Author; 1997.

ace offered current perspectives on the original guidelines, highlighting societal changes, changing professional perspectives, and challenges for updating the guidelines (Townsend, Banks, Multari, & Naugle, 1991). A growing focus in Canada on health promotion, consumer involvement, the environment, and spirituality were emphasized. Changes in professional perspectives were cited, such as occupational therapists' increasing involvement with groups, organizations, and other clients as well as individuals. Occupational therapy was also seen as awakening to its conceptual foundations, in recognizing that practice draws on phenomenology and critical social science as well as medical and other empirical sciences. The primary challenge highlighted in 1991 was "to examine how we transform our intentions to reality in everyday practice" (Townsend, Banks, Multari, & Naugle, 1991, p. ix).

CLARIFYING

The Client-Centred Practice Committee organized a Guidelines Impact Study to evaluate the original guidelines using an ethnographic design (Blain & Townsend, 1993; Blain, Townsend, Krefting, & Burwash, 1992). The purpose of the study was to

"... document how the Guidelines are being used, the usefulness of various concepts and sections, and suggestions for change in updating. Further, the study was designed to gather data on what updated guidelines ought to be like in order for them to be used and useful in the 1990s and beyond." (Blain & Townsend, 1993, p. 272)

Ethnographic data were first gathered through 21 in-depth telephone interviews with key informants, chosen by CAOT representatives and colleagues, as leaders in Canadian occupational therapy. Interview data were used to generate a survey that was distributed to a representative sample of 285 CAOT members across the country. With a response rate of 29%, the 77 people who participated were not subjects of research, but rather ethnographic informants (Blain, Townsend, Krefting, & Burwash, 1992, p. 9). Survey results showed that 81% of respondents used Volume I (1983), 44% using it as a reference at least four times per year. Volume II (1986 Intervention Guidelines) was used by 25%, and Volume III (Toward Outcome Measures, 1987) by 16% of respondents. The primary users (57%) were administrators involved in quality assurance, explaining occupational therapy to medical or health professionals, and advocacy or lobbying for clients or occupational therapy. In their conclusions, the evaluators stated

"For occupational therapy to succeed in its self-definition, updated guidelines need to articulate a clear vision of occupational therapy's own concepts, discourse and practice strategies. The vision must be one which can encompass all occupational therapists, in all areas of practice within Canada today and into the 21st century ... [it is time] to articulate a clear vision of occupational therapy's own concepts, discourse and strategies based on ideas and experiences in trying to implement client-centred practice." (Canadian Association of Occupational Therapists, 1991, p. 285)

Further evidence of the impact of the first three guidelines documents lies in the growing volume of published work on client-centred practice. For example, assessment and other stages in a client-centred process of practice have been examined (Hobson, 1996; Letts, Law, Rigby, Cooper, Stewart, & Strong, 1994; Pollock, 1993; Pollock, Baptiste, Law, McColl, Opzoomer, & Polatajko, 1993); client-centred practice has been embedded in documentation systems (Fearing, 1993; Watson, 1992); and analyses of the concepts and vision of client-centred practice have deepened understanding (Banks, 1991; Law, 1991; Law, 1995; Law, Cooper, Strong, Stewart, Rigby, & Letts, 1996; McColl, 1994; McColl & Pranger, 1994; Sherr Klein, 1995; Sumsion, 1993; Townsend, 1993; Townsend, 1996). Spirituality has received particular attention in the 1990s (Egan & DeLaat, 1994; Kirsh, 1996; Urbanowski & Vargo, 1994).

CONCENTRATING

While the impact of previous guidelines was being evaluated, *Occupational Therapy Guidelines for Client-Centred Mental Health Practice* were published (Health Canada and Canadian Association of Occupational Therapists, 1993). These are Canada's only national guidelines for a specific area, i.e., mental health practice, and were funded because mental health practice was in decline, even though psychosocial issues have been important historically in occupational therapy (Friedland & Renwick, 1993). The two main purposes of producing *Occupational Therapy Guidelines for Client-Centred Mental Health Practice* are briefly illustrated in scenarios #4 and #5.

Scenario #4: Clarifying Occupational Therapy s Role in Mental Health Services

An occupational therapist, working as a case manager on a Community Mental Health Services team, is asked to help the team justify its inclusion of occupational therapy. Referring to chapters and sections in *Occupational Therapy Guidelines for Client-Centred Mental Health Practice*, the occupational therapist describes the Occupational Performance Model, Enabling Optimal Occupational Performance, Case Management/Coordination, Occupational Therapy Mental Health Practice Roles, Guidelines for Stages of Occupational Therapy Mental Health Clinical Practice, a Practice Illustration for a Clinical Role, and Future Visions, stating that "The unique combination of knowledge about psychopathology, environmental factors and function, and the commitment to client-centred practice, means occupational therapists have an ideal set of skills for being case managers" (Health Canada and Canadian Association of Occupational Therapists, 1993, p. 19).

Scenario #5: Promoting Mental Health in all Practice Settings

Four occupational therapists who contract with a work hardening corporation are advocating for paid time to attend to the mental, as well as physical, difficulties often experienced by people with low back injuries. The corporation is reluctant to fund mental health goals in occupational therapy, claiming that most third-party insurers view mental difficulties as malingering. A Brief on Mental Health Promotion with Low Back Injuries is prepared, including a proposal for a pilot project to compare those in work hardening programmes with and without a mental health component. Referring to *Occupational Therapy Guidelines for Client-Centred Mental Health Practice*, the occupational therapists assert that "... occupational therapists view the promotion of mental health as an integral part of all occupational therapy practice" (Health Canada and Canadian Association of Occupational Therapists, 1993, p. vii).

CLASSIFYING

In a project that started in 1993, Canadian occupational therapists and Human Resources Development Canada (HRDC) undertook a unique exercise to classify competencies for client-centred practice. Functional analysis methodology was used to classify five levels of competencies in a *Profile of Occupational Therapy Practice in Canada* (Canadian Association of Occupational Therapists, 1996; Human Resources Development Canada, 1993). Representatives from diverse areas of practice across Canada were included in three stages of meetings, focus groups, and review processes. Key references were the 1991 consolidated *Occupational Therapy Guidelines for Client-Centred Practice* (Canadian Association of Occupational Therapists, 1991) and a CAOT *Position Statement on Everyday Occupations and Health* (Canadian Association of Occupational Therapists, 1994).

Functional analysis methodology had already been used in developing *Australian Competency Standards for Entry-Level Occupational Therapists* (Australian Association of Occupational Therapists, 1994). However, Canada's historical orientation to client-centred practice produced a different profile, emphasizing collaboration with clients, meaningful occupation, and occupational performance. The Canadian group classified seven Units of Professional Competency in Occupational Therapy, based on an Occupational Therapists' Key Role statement that "Occupational therapists enable individuals, groups, and communities to develop the means and opportunities to identify, engage in, and achieve desired potential in the occupations of life" (Canadian Association of Occupational Therapists, 1996, p. 82).

This Profile is now being used for developing academic standards and validating the blueprint for CAOT's National Certification Examination and occupational therapists' self assessment.

CREATING

New guidelines for client-centred practice, called *Enabling Occupation: An Occupational Therapy Perspective*, have now been published (Canadian Association of Occupational Therapists, 1997). Starting in 1993, 10 occupational therapy collaborators from clinical, administrative, and academic sites across Canada researched and wrote these guidelines based on two meetings, teleconferences, faxes, and electronic mail. Another 54 occupational therapists contributed sections or reviewed drafts between 1994 and 1996. The purpose, drawing on recommendations from the Guidelines Impact Study, was to propose concepts, processes, and outcomes for occupational therapy well into the 21st century.

Overviews of 16 contextual features provide a background for presenting occupational performance and client-centred practice as two, interrelated core concepts for enabling occupation. A new Canadian Model of Occupational Performance (CMOP) has been developed to capture the dynamic interaction between people, their environments, and their occupations over the lifespan; and principles and ethical issues for being client-centred are highlighted for clients who may be individuals, groups, agencies, or organizations. Also outlined is a process for organizing occupational therapy services, with six elements: plan services; market services; manage services; educate; access and participate in research; and evaluate services. Ten uses for these new guidelines have been proposed along with five vignettes applying these guidelines with individual clients (a child with a brain injury, a woman admitted to mental health services), organizational clients (a senior's village, a religious organization), and a legal client requiring an assessment opinion for a court case. Scenarios #6, #7, and #8 illustrate three of the 10 suggested applications.

Scenario #6: Using the Profile of Occupational Therapy Practice in Canada and Enabling Occupation: An Occupational Therapy Perspective as Companion Documents

A group of occupational therapists in a health sciences complex are asked to identify their areas of competence as part of shifting to programme management. They suggest that the key role statement in the *Profile of Occupational Therapy Practice in Canada* be used to define a mission statement and goals for occupational therapy. They also turn to *Enabling Occupation: An Occupational Therapy Perspective* for ideas on describing the context in which their competency will be reviewed, their conceptual framework for occupational performance and client-centred practice, and the seven-stage Occupational Performance Process.

Scenario #7: Documenting and Managing Client-Centred Practice

Occupational therapists in a new private practice want to ensure that they can demonstrate quality and accountability to funders and the community. They decide to document clients' priority occupational performance issues and targeted outcomes, occupational therapists' time, and costs related to each stage of the occupational performance process described in *Enabling Occupation: An Occupational Therapy Perspective*. They market their practice as *client-centred*, and organize a system of collaborative documentation in which both occupational therapists and clients record client issues, strengths and resources, targeted outcomes, plans, implementation, and evaluation. The occupational therapists and clients both use these data to speak on important local issues with the media, funding agencies, and government representatives. For accountability, the occupational therapists and clients jointly outline performance appraisal and continuing professional education.

Scenario #8: Advocating with and for Clients

Three occupational therapists who work in the same school district are committed to advocating with and for the adolescents with disabilities with whom they work. They begin their advocacy by talking with a group of adolescents, with and without disabilities, in each of their schools. To show the adolescents what they mean by being *client-centred*, they offer to support them in, but not take over, the production of posters on disability rights and inclusiveness in each school. After facilitating their separate school groups to produce posters, the occupational therapists encourage the adolescents to organize a Disability and Ability Conference involving all three schools. The posters provide a starting point for the adolescents to tell stories to students, teachers, and the media about what its like to be included or excluded from school events on the basis of ability. The occupational therapists' enabling approaches share power by involving the students in decision making, and by doing things that students choose as being appropriate to and meaningful in their adolescent culture.

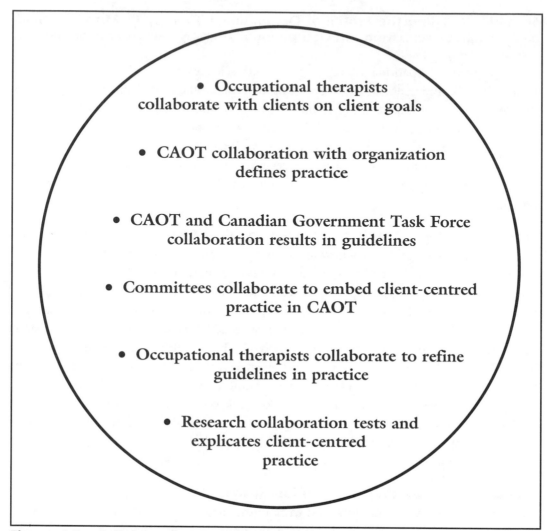

Figure 4-1. Collaboration Promoting Client-Centred Practice.

FOUR DECADES OF COLLABORATION IN DEVELOPING CANADIAN OCCUPATIONAL THERAPY GUIDELINES

From the 1960s to the end of the 1990s, many forces of collaboration, depicted in Figure 4-1, have made client-centred practice a valued, explicit, and central part of Canadian occupational therapy. Viewed as highlights in an interwoven web, a number of initiatives display the collaborative character of Canadian occupational therapy. They also illustrate how professional and government partnerships at the national level can create an environment in which collaboration is possible.

COLLABORATION IN ACTION

Three collaborative initiatives involved occupational therapists in action with clients and with those who are concerned with organizing client services. First, client-centred practice has grown because quality occupational therapy is essentially client-centred; this is a profession that works by involving clients actively. Of course, client participation in defining and pursuing meaningful outcomes may be difficult to achieve given client limitations or organizational restraints related to programme philosophy, protocols, time, and funding (Sumsion, 1993; Townsend, 1993; Townsend, 1996; Townsend, 1997). Yet, individual clients have told the profession that client-centred practice, with practical occupational outcomes, is the key to making occupational therapy a responsive and relevant profession now and into the 21st century (Sherr Klein, 1995).

A second set of initiatives, evolving through the 1960s and 1970s, saw occupational therapists collaborating directly with hospital accreditation bodies, skill profile developers, and other organizations forming definitions of practice that were based on occupational therapists' own views rather than the views of others. These organizational initiatives gave occupational therapy freedom to define an appropriate conceptual framework so that this profession can respond to the practical needs that clients present, i.e., to become client-centred and focused on occupational performance.

Third, in the 1980s and early 1990s, Canada's DNHW Clinical Guidelines Program launched a pivotal collaboration that brought together CAOT and Canadian Government interests in quality professional practice. The long-term commitment to collaboration by guidelines task force members, CAOT, and DNHW has been very important in promoting client-centred practice. CAOT initiatives, such as those described above, have included or been led by those who have been involved in client-centred guideline development for 10 to 15 years. Awareness of client-centred practice and the development of distance technology enabled task forces to collaborate with an ever-decreasing number of face-to-face meetings, from 10 for the first *Guidelines for the Client-Centred Practice of Occupational Therapy* (Department of National Health and Welfare and Canadian Association of Occupational Therapists, 1983), to two for the latest guidelines, *Enabling Occupation: A Canadian Occupational Therapy Perspective* (Canadian Association of Occupational Therapists, 1997).

COLLABORATING TO DEVELOP CLIENT-CENTRED ROUTINES

Three additional collaborative initiatives are reinforcing that client-centredness and occupational performance are routine foundations of any occupational therapy practice. For example, CAOT committees have been collaborating to make client-centred practice an official expectation in CAOT initiatives. Already, many practice papers, the National Certification Examination, accreditation standards for fieldwork and academic programs, and various policies are based on client-centred practice guidelines so that new graduates and occupational therapists who are new to Canada all routinely learn about client-centred practice and occupational performance.

A second example is that some occupational therapists have collaborated to create client-centred, occupation-focused protocols, standards, quality-management criteria, and time-management documentation for specific practice situations. For instance, the process of occupational performance described in the new guidelines for enabling occupation was adapted from work by Virginia Fearing and other occupational therapists in

Vancouver, British Columbia (Fearing, 1993). Their day-to-day collaboration, amongst themselves and with their clients, has made client-centred practice a routine expectation and an approach to documentation, not just a conceptually appealing idea. Third, there is the example of occupational therapy collaboration to test and explicate client-centred practice. Research and practice collaborations have flowed into professional arenas, such as the CAOT's Annual Conferences, where partnership and other client-centred ideas have become prominent.

REFLECTIONS ON COLLABORATION

Collaboration toward client-centred practice has been possible among occupational therapists with diverse views because Canada's Federal Clinical Guidelines Program and occupational therapists focused on illuminating core, conceptual, generic, consensus elements, and processes in occupational therapy. As a result, there has been no need to choose a particular model of practice, to create hierarchical lists of assessments or interventions that inevitably exclude or insult someone, or to take sides on specific practice issues. This generic approach has built bridges that have increased the potential for collaboration. With client-centred practice as a focus, differences in practice settings, populations, or theories have been respected with the knowledge that there are common ideas and processes that bind the profession together. Rather than battling competing forces, Canadian occupational therapists seem to have become energized by the holistic, integrated, comprehensive, socially responsive, and ultimately democratic forces that underpin client-centred practice. The emphasis on occupational performance and client-centred practice has helped to explain what makes occupational therapy a health profession in its own right. Essentially, the Canadian experience in client-centred practice has helped to empower occupational therapists to develop their own voice and vision and to enable clients to realize their visions as well.

CONCLUSION: TWO EMERGING NOTIONS OF CLIENT-CENTRED PRACTICE

After almost 40 years of collaboration, it is time to look to our future as well as our history to consider emerging notions of client-centred practice in occupational therapy. Whereas efforts in the 1960s and 1970s built a foundation for Canadian occupational therapists to take control of their own practice, the 1980s and 1990s have illuminated a direction of occupational therapy in Canada. As the 21st century approaches, two key notions about occupational therapy's client-centred practice have been captured in the new guidelines, *Enabling Occupation: An Occupational Therapy Perspective* (Canadian Association of Occupational Therapists, 1997).

One emerging notion is that occupational therapy's focus in client-centred practice is on occupation. Given that this is *occupational* therapy, it makes sense to articulate the profession's generic, conceptual framework in terms of *occupation and occupational performance*. As occupational therapists ask clients to name and prioritize their own goals, clients are naming *occupational* goals that define what they want or need to *do* to make life easier or more meaningful. Occupational therapists are realizing that client outcomes in culturally- and age-appropriate self-care, productivity, and leisure occupations must be addressed. Changes in performance components and the environment are the means to achieve these outcomes. Moreover, outcomes in self-care, productivity, and leisure occupations can be related to holistic and visionary goals for health, quality of life, empowerment, and equity. With this broader view of clients' potential, occupational therapists are emphasizing the importance of the spirit (spirituality) in achieving the occupational potential of individuals and communities. Canadian occupational therapists have debated the place of spirituality in this profession over almost 20 years and are now locating spirituality as central to the person, shaped by the environment, and giving meaning to occupations (Canadian Association of Occupational Therapists, 1997).

The other emerging notion is that client-centred practice reflects a commitment to equity and democracy. The democratic elements are that clients and occupational therapists share power as they focus on client goals and draw on client as well as professional expertise. In other words, client-centred practice brings power into view and transforms power relations. Traditional, hierarchical power relations, based on professional dominance, are challenged and shifted toward collaboration and partnership. As this happens, occupational therapy's role is shifting toward enablement. Intervention, which replaced treatment in the 1980s, is itself being replaced by phrases such as "implement plans." Increasingly, clients are asking for guidance through facilitating, mentoring, coaching, and other approaches that involve them as decision makers and problems solvers in their own lives or organizations. Enablement draws occupational therapists to attend to the context of their practice and clients' experiences and to challenge the appropriateness of standardized protocols, which may negate individual and contextual differences. The emergence of client-centred practice, then, is enabling occupational therapists and clients to advocate for relationships that are mutually empowering.

REFERENCES

Australian Association of Occupational Therapists (1994). *Australian competency standards for entry-level occupational therapists.* Sydney: Author.

Banks, S. (1991). The Canadian model of occupational performance: Its relevance to community practice. *Canadian Journal of Occupational Therapy, 58,* 109-111.

Blain, J., & Townsend, E. (1993). Occupational therapy guidelines for client-centred practice: Impact study findings. *Canadian Journal of Occupational Therapy, 60,* 271-285.

Blain, J., Townsend, E., Krefting, L., & Burwash, S. (1992). *Occupational therapy guidelines for client-centred practice: Impact study evaluation and recommendations.* Toronto, ON: CAOT Publications.

Bridle, M. J. (1977). Profile of an occupational therapist: A report on the project to date. *Canadian Journal of Occupational Therapy, 45,* 23-26.

Bridle, M. J. (1981). Profile of an occupational therapist revisited. *Canadian Journal of Occupational Therapy, 48,* 107-113.

Canadian Association of Occupational Therapists (1991). *Occupational therapy guidelines for client-centred practice.* Toronto, ON: CAOT Publications.

Canadian Association of Occupational Therapists (1994). Position statement on everyday occupations and health. *Canadian Journal of Occupational Therapy, 61,* 294-297.

Canadian Association of Occupational Therapists (1996). Profile of occupational therapy practice in Canada. *Canadian Journal of Occupational Therapy, 63,* 79-113.

Canadian Association of Occupational Therapists (1997). *Enabling occupation: An occupational therapy perspective.* Ottawa, ON: CAOT Publications.

Canadian Council for Health Services Accreditation (1995). *Standards for rehabilitation organizations: A client-centred approach.* Ottawa, ON: Author.

Canadian Council on Hospital Accreditation (1977). *Guide to hospital accreditation.* Toronto, ON: Author.

Department of National Health and Welfare and Canadian Association of Occupational Therapists (1983). *Guidelines for the client-centred practice of occupational therapy.* Ottawa, ON: Minister of Supply and Services Canada, Cat. No. H39-33/1983E.

Department of National Health and Welfare and Canadian Association of Occupational Therapists (1986). *Intervention guidelines for the client-centred practice of occupational therapy.* Ottawa, ON: Minister of Supply and Services Canada, Cat. No. H39-100/1986E.

Donabedian, A. (1966). Evaluating the quality of medical care. *Milbank Memorial Fund Quarterly, 44, Suppl.,* 166-206.

Egan, M., & DeLaat, M. D. (1994). Considering spirituality in occupational therapy practice. *Canadian Journal of Occupational Therapy, 61,* 95-101.

Fearing, V. G. (1993). Occupational therapists chart a course through the health record. *Canadian Journal of Occupational Therapy, 60,* 232-240.

Friedland, J., & Renwick, R. M. (1993). The issue is—Psychosocial occupational therapy: Time to cast off the gloom and doom. *American Journal of Occupational Therapy, 47,* 467-471.

Health Canada and Canadian Association of Occupational Therapists. (1993). *Occupational therapy guidelines for client-centred mental health practice.* Ottawa, ON: Minister of Supply and Services.

Hobson, S. (1996). Being client-centred when the client is cognitively impaired. *Canadian Journal of Occupational Therapy, 63,* 133-137.

Human Resources Development Canada (1993). *Support materials on functional analysis approach.* Toronto, ON.

Kirsh, B. (1996). A narrative approach to addressing spirituality in occupational therapy: Exploring personal meaning and purpose. *Canadian Journal of Occupational Therapy, 63,* 55-61.

Law, M. (1991). Muriel Driver memorial lecture: The environment: A focus for occupational therapy. *Canadian Journal of Occupational Therapy, 58,* 171-180.

Law, M. (1995). Client-centred practice: What does it mean and does it make a difference? *Canadian Journal of Occupational Therapy, 62,* 250-257.

Law, M., Baptiste, S., Carswell, A., McColl, M. A., Polatajko, H., & Pollock, N. (1994). *Canadian occupational performance measure,* (2nd ed.). Toronto, ON: CAOT Publications ACE.

Law, M., Baptiste, S., McColl, M. A., Opzoomer, A., Polatajko, H., & Pollock, N. (1990). The Canadian Occupational Performance Measure: An outcome measure for occupational therapy. *Canadian Journal of Occupational Therapy, 57,* 82-87.

Law, M., Cooper, B., Strong, S., Stewart, D., Rigby, P., & Letts, L. (1996). The person-environment-occupation model: A transactive approach to occupational performance. *Canadian Journal of Occupational Therapy, 63,* 9-23.

Letts, L., Law, M., Rigby, P., Cooper, B., Stewart, D., & Strong, S. (1994). Person-environment assessments in occupational therapy. *American Journal of Occupational Therapy, 48,* 608-618.

Management Information Systems Group (1993). *Guidelines for management information systems in Canadian health care facilities: Diagnostic and therapeutic services—Occupational therapy manual.* Ottawa, ON: Author.

McColl, M. A. (1994). Holistic occupational therapy: Historical meaning and contemporary implications. *Canadian Journal of Occupational Therapy, 61,* 72-77.

McColl, M. A., & Pranger, T. (1994). Theory and practice in the occupational therapy guidelines for client-centred practice. *Canadian Journal of Occupational Therapy, 61,* 250-259.

Pollock, N. (1993). Client-centred assessment. *American Journal of Occupational Therapy, 47,* 298-301.

Pollock, N., Baptiste, S., Law, M., McColl, M. A., Opzoomer, A., & Polatajko, H. (1993). Occupational performance measures: A review based on the guidelines for the client-centred practice of occupational therapy. *Canadian Journal of Occupational Therapy, 57,* 77-81.

Reed, K., & Sanderson, S. R. (1980). *Concepts of occupational therapy.* Baltimore: Williams and Wilkins.

Sherr Klein, B. S. (1995). Reflections ... An ally as well as a partner in practice. *Canadian Journal of Occupational Therapy, 62,* 283-285.

Sumsion, T. (1993). Client-centred practice: The true impact. *Canadian Journal of Occupational Therapy, 60,* 6-8.

Townsend, E. A. (1993). Muriel Driver memorial lecture: Occupational therapy's social vision. *Canadian Journal of Occupational Therapy, 60,* 174-184.

Townsend, E. A. (1996). Enabling empowerment: Using simulations versus real occupations. *Canadian Journal of Occupational Therapy, 63,* 114-128.

Townsend, E. A. (1997). *Good intentions overruled: A critique of empowerment in the routine organization of mental health services.* Toronto, ON: University of Toronto Press.

Townsend, E., Banks, S., Multari, L., & Naugle, A. (1991). Preface to the 1991 Edition: Current perspectives on the original guidelines. In Canadian Association of Occupational Therapists. *Occupational therapy guidelines for client-centred practice.* Toronto, ON: CAOT Publications, pp. v-ix.

Townsend, E., Brintnell, S., & Staisey, N. (1990). Developing guidelines for client-centred occupational therapy practice. *Canadian Journal of Occupational Therapy, 57,* 69-76.

Townsend, E., Ryan, B., & Law, M. (1990). Using the World Health Organization's International Classification of Impairments, Disabilities, and Handicaps in Occupational Therapy. *Canadian Journal of Occupational Therapy, 57,* 16-25.

Trent, M. (1919). Story beyond the badge. *The Vocational Bulletin. Department of Soldiers Civil Reestablishment, June,* 2-5.

Urbanowski, R., & Vargo, J. (1994). Spirituality, daily practice, and the Occupational Performance Model. *Canadian Journal of Occupational Therapy, 61,* 88 94.

Watson, D. (1992). Documentation of paediatric assessments using the occupational therapy guidelines for client-centred practice. *Canadian Journal of Occupational Therapy, 59,* 87-94.

THE CLIENT-CENTRED OCCUPATIONAL THERAPY PROCESS

VIRGINIA G. FEARING, BSc, OT(C), JO CLARK, BSc, OT(C),
SUE STANTON, MA, OT(C)

Occupational therapy is grounded in principles and values that honour the rights and potential of every client, whether that client is a corporation, community, group, or an individual. These principles are reflected in every thoughtful interaction between therapist and client. At its best, occupational therapy is an apparently simple process that helps clients make order and meaning out of complex and challenging situations. This deceptively simple process is, in fact, multidimensional, collaborative, and creative. It enables clients to envision their futures to the extent that they are willing to work toward them. This means that the worked-for future must have meaning and value to individual clients.

Occupational therapists have long been vocal in their belief that the client is central to the occupational therapy process. Transforming that belief into everyday practice requires therapists to exhibit client-centred behaviours that are recognizable by others, especially the client. As clients respond, both client and therapist behaviours become indicators of client-centred interactions. For example, ensuring that clients have enough information can result in clients making informed decisions. However, although these behaviours are healthy indicators, they do not guarantee that the occupational therapy process will flow in a logical and client-centred way.

Fearing, Law, and Clark (1997) have described an Occupational Performance Process Model (OPPM) that provides a client-centred, flexible, yet focused, framework to guide the therapist and client through seven stages of collaborative, outcome-oriented process (Figure 5-1). This model, which focuses on resolving occupational performance issues, makes it possible for the client to continue in the process, regardless of the setting or therapist. The following discussion of the OPPM includes client and therapist behaviours that may be viewed as indicators of client-centred practice. Key therapist behaviours are highlighted in the text.

OCCUPATIONAL PERFORMANCE PROCESS MODEL

In stage 1, the therapist and client name, validate, and prioritize occupational performance issues. Therapists who practice from a client-centred stance recognize that, in order to resolve occupational performance issues, more than one client may be involved. For example, potential clients include a premature baby and its parents, the staff as well

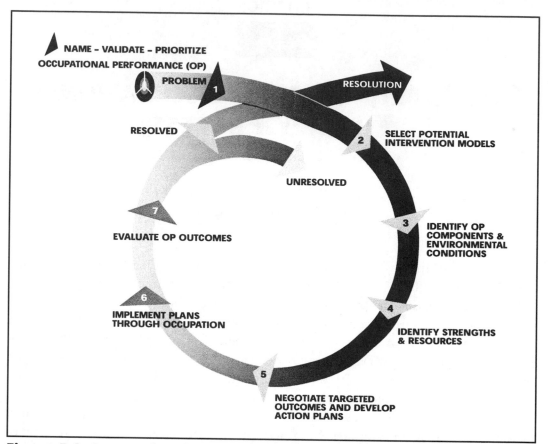

Figure 5-1. Occupational Performance Process Model. Fearing, V., Law, M., and Clark, J. (1997). Reprinted with permission of the *Canadian Journal of Occupational Therapy*.

as executives in a company, the caregivers and the person with Alzheimer's disease, workers and the organization trying to return those workers to the workforce. Occupational therapists view each client as inseparable from a unique context (Mattingly, 1991). When beginning the occupational therapy process, they include not only the primary client, but also associated clients who contribute to and are affected by resolution of the issues raised.

> Include associated clients.

Stage 1 is the screening part of the process. Its purpose is to identify whether or not there are occupational performance issues that are important to the client. The occupational therapist asks the client to talk about self-care, productivity, and leisure performance.

> Ask the client to talk about occupational performance issues.

This client narrative is critically important not only to identify issues, but also to place those issues within each client's unique temporal, physical, environmental, and social context. The information that comes from narrative is far different from information gathered from a checklist method of identifying client issues.

The occupational therapist listens carefully and then reflects back to the client the issues that are identified during the narrative.

> ## Listen carefully. Reflect back.

The therapist invites the client to make changes to the list of issues to ensure that it is a true reflection of the client's concerns.

> ## Validate occupational performance issues.

Once the issues are identified and the client has validated them, the occupational therapist asks the client to rank them in order of priority to the client. A standard method is this uses the Canadian Occupational Performance Measure (Law, et al., 1994).

> ## Client sets occupational performance priorities.

If there are no actual or potential occupational performance issues, the occupational therapist explains to the client that the occupational therapy process will not benefit the client as there are no identified occupational performance issues. The therapist may advocate by linking the client to other necessary contacts.

> ## Advocate.

However, when there are occupational performance issues that are important to the client, and the client is ready to work on them, the therapist seeks client permission to initiate assessment to identify the causes of the issues.

In stage 2, the therapist selects potential intervention models to use in gathering information about the components and environmental conditions that are contributing to the occupational performance issues. McColl, Law, and Stewart (1993) have developed a useful classification system for theory that can assist the therapist in thinking about the selection of appropriate assessments and interventions. Remaining current in research-based approaches enables the therapist to creatively use appropriate approaches to guide reasoning during the process.

> ## Use appropriate theoretical approaches.

For example, depending on the client's occupational performance issues and contributing components and environments, the therapist may use a biomechanical approach from the physical-rehabilitative category as well as theories about grief and loss from the psycho-emotional category, and role change from the socio-adaptive category when assessing the issues identified by one client. Use of more than one approach is common. Therapists who have specialized to the extent that they can use only one theoretical approach must be extremely careful not to limit the client's options to match the therapist's ability, or lack of ability.

Critically review approaches and new research.

In keeping with the idea of advocacy, occupational therapists recognize and act on their need to receive coaching or assistance in order to address client issues; for example, a therapist seeks feedback from others when developing competence in using an unfamiliar theoretical approach. Referral to another agency or therapist may be necessary to ensure that the client's therapist has the knowledge and skills to address the client's issues. Once theoretical approaches have been identified, the therapist selects appropriate assessment tools to gather further information and revisits these theories when planning intervention.

In stage 3, guided by the theoretical approaches identified during stage 2, the therapist and client identify occupational performance components and environmental conditions contributing to the issues that were identified in stage 1. An occupational performance issue identified during stage 1, for example inability to go outside unaccompanied, might have the following component identified during assessment: unable to find her way. Another person might have the same occupational performance issue, inability to go outside unaccompanied, but completely different components and environmental conditions contributing to that issue; for example, steps from home are slippery and unsafe. The therapist makes no assumptions but checks out information with the clients involved.

Focus on facts. Avoid judgments and assumptions.

In stage 4, the therapist and client identify strengths and resources. In addition to client strengths, caregiver, community, therapist, and environmental resources are important to the successful resolution of identified issues. Occupational therapists consider clients to be experts regarding their own situations and their usual methods for problem solving (Canadian Association of Occupational Therapists, 1996). Using these unique strategies and resources in the plan makes it relevant to the client's everyday experience.

An important part of the occupational therapy process is enabling clients to enhance their problem-solving skills.

Value the client as an expert.

The client-therapist partnership is a significant resource. The occupational therapist considers the extent to which it is possible to collaborate in a therapist-client partnership that will meet the client's needs. For example, even if the risk-taking styles of the therapist and client differ, the therapist's task is to decide whether this client's risk-taking behaviour is a matter of personal style or a lack of competent judgment (Hobson, 1996).

> ### Respect differences in opinion or style.

Therapists in a client-centred process become highly tuned to their role as facilitator, working with every resource available, whether or not the therapist personally has, or values, those same resources. When the therapist and client cannot collaborate effectively, or the client does not feel comfortable working with the therapist, another therapist is identified for the client. Such matching to facilitate an optimal client-therapist partnership is a common practice in professions. The occupational therapist reflects on the information gathered, considering client values and usual methods for addressing issues.

> ### Use strengths and resources.

Paradoxically, therapists who practice from a client-centred stance become empowered themselves. While focusing on a client-centred process, therapists cannot ignore barriers to client progress and so the therapist-advocate is born and becomes another resource.

In stage 5, the therapist and client negotiate targeted outcomes and develop action plans. A targeted outcome is an agreed upon and measurable performance at a given time in the future toward which to work.

> ### Imagine a possible client future.

The therapist and client look ahead and envision a possible client future. They identify targeted outcomes related to the occupational performance issues identified in stage 1. In order to resolve these issues, the client and therapist take action and address the components or environmental conditions contributing to those issues. The occupational therapist ensures that clients have the necessary information to make informed decisions.

> ### Share information.

In this process, the occupational therapist keeps no secrets. This promotes client trust in the therapist and in the process. As they become active players in the process, clients generally assume more responsibility for their health. They are more likely to speak up for themselves, to relax and laugh, and to make suggestions.

Sometimes therapists may avoid or discourage the client's vision of the future. Perhaps the client's wishes are viewed as unattainable, whether from service mandate, available resources, or a misfit between therapist and client viewpoints. During the occupational performance process, both client and therapist may gain more insight into strengths and limitations, choosing to maintain the original course or refocusing energy in another direction. Believing in clients gives a strong message about the degree to which clients can begin to believe in themselves. Building bridges to the future, not barriers, is the focus of the occupational therapist even if it may require a leap of faith.

Once targeted outcomes are agreed upon, and the initial action plan has been established, as with any contract, it is important to identify responsibilities of each person involved.

Clarify action plan and responsibilities.

The occupational therapist facilitates clarification of the actions to be taken by all involved in the process. The partners in this process may build into their action plans an agreement to laugh, to share emotions, to alleviate fear and anxiety, and to celebrate outcomes and life, through simple ceremony.

In stage 6, the plans made in stage 5 are implemented through occupation.

Because both client and therapist are clear about the targeted outcome, they can be flexible with the methods they use to achieve that outcome.

Be flexible in choosing methods to reach targets.

The occupational therapist coaches clients to become more and more active in the problem-solving process. Clients who understand the relationship of the planned actions to their issues are likely to follow those plans or substitute an activity that is equally effective.

Coach clients.

Putting away groceries may achieve physical objectives and also have occupational meaning to a client who must work in a kitchen. Stacking cones to improve hand coordination may achieve physical objectives, but be without occupational meaning to the client. Clients need to recognize graded activities as steps toward desired outcomes. In a client-centred occupational therapy process, clients experience satisfaction in the process of achieving their desired targets. Celebrating before rushing on to the next challenging task is one means of gaining energy.

In stage 7, the therapist and client evaluate occupational performance outcomes. Throughout the process, there is ongoing comparison between targeted outcomes and current performance. At any stage in the process, the therapist and client may circle back to the beginning of the process and refocus direction. In stage 7, the client has come full circle to the beginning of the process when the occupational performance issues of importance to the client were initially identified. Sometimes targeted outcomes are achieved in their entirety. Resolution of one set of issues may create other issues that need to be addressed. These new issues are addressed through the seven-stage process, just as the original issues were. At other times, targeted outcomes are partially achieved, or portions of the outcome are reached in different settings.

Document outcomes.

The partnership that sets achievable expected outcomes and leaves documented evidence of progress makes it easy for the client to continue along the agreed upon process even if the therapists change.

Sometimes, targeted outcomes are not achieved at all. In this case, or when the results are puzzling, the occupational therapist and client review the seven-stage process to identify where the process went astray.

Review process and make necessary changes.

The data collected from comparing targeted outcomes to actual outcomes can be very valuable to the client and also provides information to the therapist about practice on a daily basis. It is important to know which issues are effectively addressed and which are not. For those issues that are not resolved, what different interventions might have resulted in a better outcome? The occupational therapist responds to evidence gathered during evaluation by changing practice where there is evidence to support change.

EXAMPLES

The following four examples demonstrate the occupational performance process with a client who does not require occupational therapy, a client in the home setting who completes the process for one issue and will continue to use the process for other issues, a client with mental health issues (Table 5-5), who completes the process, and a client in an industrial setting who completes the process. These examples are simplified to focus on process and client-centred behaviour.

EXAMPLE 1

Stage 1: Name, Validate, and Prioritize Occupational Performance Issues

In the initial interview, the therapist uses an assessment tool, the Canadian Occupational Performance Measure (COPM) (Law, Baptiste, Carswell-Opzoomer, McColl, Polatajko, & Pollock, 1994), to enable the client to paint a picture of what her life looks like given her chronic pain. Lisa describes having previously completed numerous assessments at the pain clinic where she received pain medication and learned a number of pain management and relaxation techniques. She finds all of these very helpful, but I still have pain. The therapist asks questions about the things that Lisa might not be able to do as well as she used to, and about how the pain is manifesting itself in her lifestyle. Lisa responds,

> Well ... I decided a couple of years ago that I wasn t going to let this pain interfere with my life. When I was at the pain clinic, they taught me a number of ways to adapt activities, schedule and pace myself so I don t overdo it, and use positioning and relaxation techniques to lessen the pain. So, I wouldn t say that it interferes with my ability to do things. In fact, working part-time and having two

kids who are coming into their teens means that I have to be active. I just find that at times the pain causes me to feel more irritable. So, either I have more con-flict with my family or it takes a lot of energy to keep it at bay."

The therapist paraphrases Lisa's concerns, "You seem to be saying that, at this time, the primary issues are pain tolerance and the effect pain has on your relationships with your family." If Lisa agrees that this is an accurate reflection of her issues, then validation has occurred, and the process continues. If she says that it is not an accurate reflection, then the issues must be restated until they accurately reflect Lisa's concerns.

The therapist comments that Lisa's continued use of the techniques appears to be working well for her. Because one of the presenting issues is pain tolerance, which Lisa has already stated is being addressed, the outstanding issue is episodic conflict with fam-ily that may be viewed as a component rather than an occupational performance issue. The occupational therapist considers what profession would best serve Lisa's needs and shares recommendations with Lisa for her consideration.

This example demonstrates that by naming, validating, and prioritizing occupational performance issues, the therapist and client maintain focus on occupational performance issues that matter to the client. When components are not related to any occupational performance issues, the client and therapist consider other resources and initiate referral as necessary. Thus, with some clients, the occupational performance process ends after stage 1. The client-centred behaviours observed are client narration, reflection, valida-tion, and advocacy.

EXAMPLE 2

Stage 1: Name, Validate, and Prioritize Occupational Performance Issues

In the initial interview, the occupational therapist meets with both Mr. and Mrs. Tilly in their home. Mrs. Tilly begins her story by expressing frustration with her husband's condition.

"You have to understand ... the man we see today is not the same person who was looking forward to retirement a year ago. He used to be so active, but now he seems to have just given up. He's only 64, and I'm only 60! He had two strokes, the first one 8 months ago and the last one only 4 months ago. Now, our lives have changed because of the weakness on his left side. It's so difficult. I'm still working part-time at the cafeteria, and our sons help out, but it's so much work, and they have their own families. Before he left the hospital, they set us up with a homemaker. She tries to come when I'm at work (3 days a week) and helps him with his bathing, because we were having trouble with that. The depressing part is that he just sits around and watches television all day. We encourage him to do as much as he can, but this has really affected his spirit. He is becoming angrier and more critical of everything we do. He was never like that before."

The therapist encourages Mr. and Mrs. Tilly to continue describing how the strokes have affected or changed their lifestyles. Mr. Tilly reports that he had retired (he was previously employed as an electrician) just one year before his first stroke. Now, due to the left hemiplegia he feels useless and "a burden" to his family.

"I really enjoy the outdoors; I used to fish a lot and looked forward to doing more of it in my retirement. Now, I can't drive myself up to the lake or even hold the fishing rod when I get there. My wife has driven me up there a couple of times, but she's bored and I feel like a burden to her. This has been unfair to me, but most unfair to my wife. I get angry and take it out on her, which is even worse. We had planned to travel after she retired, and now I worry about that. I don't want her to be tied down with me. She is already doing so much extra work, I can't ask her to drive me around to do things."

Mr. Tilly went on to describe himself as having "cabin fever."

"I tried going to a senior's centre. The adapted bus came to pick me up, but when I got to the centre, they put me in some pottery and painting classes. I didn't have enough hand control, and half the time I couldn't even get the tops off the paint tubes so I just quit going."

Mr. Tilly reports he is able to get around the house to some degree with the use of a cane and foot drop splint; however, he continues to have difficulty on uneven surfaces or outdoors. He no longer drives the car due to perceptual and motor difficulties. This dramatically affects his leisure activities. It also affects banking and shopping, which have now been delegated to his wife and sons. He can prepare light meals for himself during the day, but continues to have difficulty with activities that require two hands, such as cutting food. He dresses and grooms himself, although slowly, and he receives assistance with bathing from the homemaker.

Mr. Tilly also expresses feelings of loss over occupations such as outdoor and indoor maintenance of their home. He had several post-retirement projects that he is now unable to complete. Mrs. Tilly states that their sons are providing a lot of support in this area. They frequently spend weekends and free time finishing off these projects and maintaining the lawns and gardens. "I know they are being helpful, and I appreciate it," Mr. Tilly responded, "but I feel guilty. They have lives and families of their own. They can't continue this forever."

Before recording the above information in the related areas of self-care, productivity, and leisure on the Canadian Occupational Performance Measure form (Law, Baptiste, Carswell-Opzoomer, McColl, Polatajko, & Pollock, 1994), the therapist validates the Tillys' issues by paraphrasing their concerns as lack of quality leisure activity (fishing, travel), slowness in dressing and grooming, inability to bathe independently, inability to drive and consequent changes in banking and shopping roles and leisure routines, difficulty cutting food, and inability to do home, lawn, and garden maintenance (currently undertaken by their sons). The Tillys verified that this was correct and were then asked to prioritize their concerns.

Table 5-1
Example 2: Client identified occupational performance issues

Stage 1: Client identified OP issues	Performance	Satisfaction
#1 Limited mobility in the community	1	1
#2 Lack of stimulating leisure occupations	1	2
#3 Unable to tend lawn and gardens	1	1

The three occupational performance issues rated as highest in importance by the Tillys were limited mobility in the community, lack of stimulating leisure occupations, and inability to tend to the lawn and gardens (see Table 5-1). The Tillys wanted to work on these issues first, as they held most significance in their lifestyles.

Using the COPM, the client ranks each identified occupational performance issue on a scale for performance from 1 (not able to do at all) to 10 (able to do extremely well), and a scale for satisfaction from 1 (not satisfied at all) to 10 (extremely satisfied).

Stage 2: Select Potential Intervention Models

The therapist considers what approaches to take in selecting assessments and chooses the following theoretical categories: neuro-integrative and physical rehabilitative to understand and direct physical rehabilitation; psychosocial to understand and guide adjustment to the illness experience; and environmental to understand adaptations.

Stage 3: Identify Occupational Performance Components and Environmental Conditions

Further evaluation (using a number of assessments) identifies performance components and environmental conditions (Table 5-2) contributing to the occupational performance issues. These are validated by the clients, just as the occupational performance issues were, to ensure that they are correct. Table 5-2 includes both the occupational performance issues and their contributing components and environments.

Stage 4: Identify Strengths and Resources

Mr. and Mrs. Tilly have many internal strengths and resources, some they have not yet used.

- Mrs. Tilly is involved and supportive. Both children assist with driving, household repairs, and upkeep, and will stay with Mr. Tilly if Mrs. Tilly wants to get away to visit her sister and family.
- The Tillys have many friends. Mr. Tilly has a strong relationship with his grandson who lives nearby.
- Mrs. Tilly tends to be quite positive and energetic, encouraging Mr. Tilly to do as much as he can, frequently taking him out to leisure activities with the family.
- They are currently very happy with their homemaking services.

Table 5-2
Example 2: Client identified occupational performance issues and components

---

Stage 1: Client identified OP issues and Stage 3: Components

#1 Limited mobility in the community related to: inability to drive, unsteady balance & gait on uneven surfaces, lack of awareness of resources, Mr. Tilly's reluctance to rely on family and friends.

#2 Lack of stimulating leisure occupations related to: inability to drive self or use bus due to remote location (fishing), inability to stabilize fishing rod with L hand, inability to prepare hook and rod assembly with one hand.

#3 Unable to tend lawn and gardens related to: inability to get down stairs, unsteady balance and gait on uneven surfaces, experiences general fatigue after 30 minutes, lack of awareness of energy conservation and work simplification techniques.

- They are financially stable and secure.
- Mrs. Tilly is physically able and healthy, so that she has been able to undertake some of the roles that Mr. Tilly is currently unable to resume.
- The therapist is able to contribute expertise in the areas of occupational analysis, skill development possibilities, and adaptation related to person, occupation, or environment.

Stage 5: Negotiate Targeted Outcomes and Develop Action Plans

Using the data collected in stages 1 and 3, and considering the resources identified in stage 4, the Tillys and the therapist now plan therapeutic goals and the path they wish to take to achieve them. They agree on a targeted outcome and target date toward which to work, and identify each person's role in achieving that outcome.

In Table 5-3, one of the issues, lack of stimulating leisure activities, will be used as an example.

Stage 6: Implement Plans Through Occupation

In keeping with the action plan in stage 5, the Tillys and the therapist now engage in various occupations to work toward Mr. Tilly's goal related to fishing. The therapist considers occupations that have meaning and purpose to the Tillys. This contributes to their understanding of the problem-solving process and makes it easier for them to assume responsibility. For example, after viewing the river bank with the occupational therapist and selecting the most negotiable route (in keeping with environmental theories), Mr. Tilly understands that he will need to improve his standing balance and walk down a 4-foot decline with the assistance of one person (neuro-integrative and physical rehabilita-

Table 5-3
Example 2: Client issues, components,
targeted outcomes and action plans

Stage 1: Client identified OP issues and Stage 3: Components	Stage 5: Client targeted outcomes	Stage 5: Action plans
#2 Lack of stimulating leisure occupations related to: inability to drive self or use bus due to remote location (fishing,) inability to stabilize fishing rod with L hand, inability to prepare hook and rod assembly with one hand.	To get to the local lake with companion and enjoy 3-4 hours of fishing within the next 2 months.	**Mr. & Mrs. Tilly**: contact previous fishing buddies, fishing clubs/associations regarding a companion to provide transportation and social support. **Mr. Tilly**: talk to his teenage grandson who is also interested in fishing, and teach him to tie flies and prepare a number of hook-ups in advance. He may also ask him to join the fishing trips. **Mr. Tilly & Therapist**: visit fishing locations to assess physical environment (access issues) and work towards increasing balance on uneven surfaces. Visit fishing stores and look at fishing rod apparatus regarding opportunity to adapt for one-handed purposes. Explore and learn energy conservation and work simplification techniques.

tive theories). Thus, the use of balance and tolerance exercises daily now have significant meaning and motivation, as they occur within the context of a desired occupation. Throughout this implementation stage, the therapist and the Tillys gather information, monitor progress related to changes in person, occupation, or environment (Law, Cooper, Strong, Stewart, Rigby, & Letts, 1996), collaborate, and prepare to alter or change the course as needed to meet their destination. At times, unanticipated barriers or obstacles may arise. For example, Mr. Tilly and the therapist found themselves becoming access advocates when, in the middle of their plan, the municipality decided to close off the route Mr. Tilly took to the lake.

Stage 7: Evaluate Occupational Performance Outcomes

As Mr. Tilly has now resolved to his satisfaction (and Mrs. Tilly's) one of the three occupational performance issues he identified (Table 5-4), they can now go through the same seven-stage problem-solving process to deal with the remaining issues. The Tillys are thrilled with the results so far and want to continue resolving outstanding occupational performance concerns. The therapist plans to coach them as they increase their ability to problem solve issues that are important to them.

This case illustrates problem resolution in response to a client's unique situation. It also demonstrates the power of believing in the client. From the beginning, Mrs. Tilly and the therapist actively supported Mr. Tilly's target of getting to the lake he had previously fished. Creative measures must be undertaken not only to respond to individual needs, but to break down walls and build bridges to attain client outcomes.

EXAMPLE 3

The seven-stage process of client-centred occupational therapy practice works equally well across various age groups, therapeutic settings, and predominant barriers or obstacles to functioning. Table 5-5 is an example of the same seven-stage process with a client experiencing mental health issues and psychosocial conditions that interfere with occupational performance.

EXAMPLE 4

Stage 1: Name, Validate, and Prioritize Occupational Performance Issues

The occupational therapist meets with Bob Shelley, the vice-president of a large food distribution company, and Ted Clifton and Andy Thompson who are the heads of shipping and receiving, respectively. At the outset of the meeting, Bob indicates that the occupational therapist has been consulted "to find out why the injury rate among warehouse staff in shipping and receiving has been increasing over the past 6 months." He adds, "The company is concerned about the men who are injured, as well as the effect of the injuries on business, and the workload and performance of other workers." Ted and Andy agree. Ted expresses concern about their staff.

"Two men have been on sick leave for 2 months after getting injured here. Since they left, other workers have been off sick more often. It seems that as more and more workers are off sick, either for a few days or longer, the pressure on those working increases."

Table 5-4

Example 2: Client issues, components, targeted outcomes and outcomes

Stage 1: Client identified OP issues and Stage 3: Components	Stage 5: Client targeted outcomes	Stage 7: Evaluate occupational performance outcomes
#2 Lack of stimulating leisure occupations related to: inability to drive self or use bus due to remote location (fishing), inability to stabilize fishing rod with L hand, inability to prepare hook and rod assembly with one hand.	To get to the local lake with companion and enjoy 3-4 hours of fishing within the next 2 months.	With modifications to his fishing rod, assistance and companionship from a friend and his grandson, and linkup with the local fishing club for transportation, Mr. Tilly is able to participate in weekly 3 hour fishing trips within 3 weeks of the onset of the plan. Reassessment using the C.O.P.M. demonstrated the following changes: O.P.Issue #2: lack of stimulating leisure occupations. COPM performance score changed from 1 to 7 (60% improvement) and the satisfaction score changed from 2 to 9 (70% improvement).

Andy comments on the impact of this for the department.

"We have noticed that orders are being filled late, and there are increased reports from clients of order errors and damaged goods. We are aware that this situation is stressful for staff but it is also not good for business. I think that reducing or eliminating the injuries would rectify this situation."

The occupational therapist seeks clarification, "So, your underlying concern then is the potential injury of other workers in the shipping and receiving departments?"

"Not only that," Bob responds, "we also want to identify why the injuries are occurring so the injured workers do not re-injure themselves when they return to work."

Table 5-5

Example 3: Elisabeth is a 56 y/o single, female living alone in an urban area. She has been admitted to an acute, in-patient mental health unit due to a depressive episode of a long standing bipolar illness.

Stage 1: Client identified OP issues	Stage 2: Potential intervention models	Stage 3: Components and conditions	Stage 4: Client identified strengths and resources	Stage 5: Client targeted outcomes	Stage 6: Implementation of plans through occupation	Stage 7: Evaluate outcomes
1) "I'm not sure I can live on my own anymore. I had decompensated so much I wasn't eating and rarely got out of bed- although I wasn't sleeping either." Performance 1/10 (COPM) Satisfaction 1/10 (COPM) 2) "I've cut myself off from everything. I used to see friends, volunteer, garden. but now I feel I have nothing." Performance 2/10 Satisfaction 1/10	• Social learning • Behavioural • Cognitive-Behavioural • Environmental	• decreased physical stamina and tolerance • lacks techniques to manage hand tremor (medication side effect) • feels overwhelmed and incapable • perceives self as a burden to others and thinks friends are disappointed and angry with her • feels anxious in social situations • has discontinued contact with friends and social connections as well as professional supports and resources over the past 6 months	• "I used to have a strong support network" • "I'm well travelled and love to share my experiences with others" • "I've done a lot of volunteer work, helping others seems to help me feel good about myself"	• To return to living at home independently • To reconnect with friends and social supports • To develop and pursue at least two new leisure pursuits in the community which will help to expand her personal network	• home visit to establish current baseline of self care skills and begin the process of problem solving, skill-building and adaptation • cognitive restructuring techniques to challenge unbalanced perceptions of self • use relaxation techniques to engage in social activities with a minimum amount of anxiety • leisure interest and needs inventory • explore local community resources and link up with at least 2 resources prior to discharge	OP issue #1: Ability to live independently related to meal preparation & personal care. Performance: 7/10 (60% improvement) Satisfaction: 8/10 (70% improvement) OP issue #2: Reconnection with friends and two additional leisure pursuits: Performance: 8/10 (60% improvement) Satisfaction: 10/10 (90% improvement)

The occupational therapist recognizes one occupational performance issue from Bob, Ted, and Andy's narrative descriptions: Potential for new injuries and/or recurring injuries among workers in the shipping and receiving departments. The therapist asks Bob, Ted, and Andy if this statement accurately reflects their concerns. They agree, validating the occupational performance issue. Because it is the only issue, it has priority.

The occupational therapist asks Ted and Andy to briefly describe the tasks and activities that the warehouse staff carry out in a typical day to enhance her understanding of their work and enable her to judge whether occupational therapy services might benefit the company. Ted responds,

"The workers do a number of different jobs depending on what is required. They pick the orders, load product on to pallets, sometimes they stretch-wrap the pallets when they come off the production line, move the pallets around the warehouse using forklift trucks, and haul the doors up and down when orders are shipped. They do a lot of lifting."

Andy adds, "they do similar things in my department, but instead of getting orders ready to go out, they deal with goods that are received."

The therapist reasons that a variety of personal factors (occupational performance components) and environmental factors could be contributing to the occupational performance issue and decides that the company could benefit from occupational therapy services. She facilitates a discussion that leads to an occupational therapy contract with the company in which the occupational therapist will provide the following services in sequence:

- Identify the factors that are contributing to the work injuries by interviewing current staff in the shipping and receiving departments and staff on leave, and observing warehouse staff carrying out tasks and activities associated with their work.
- Make recommendations about changes that are needed to reduce the likelihood of injury to workers.
- Provide a full written report of the findings and recommendations.
- Present the recommendations verbally to management and staff representatives.

Bob comments, "I hope that we will be able to negotiate an additional contract to address any concerns that are identified, once this first stage is complete."

Stage 2: Identify Potential Intervention Models

The therapist considers the possible theoretical approaches that could guide the choice of assessments and selects approaches from the physical, rehabilitative, and environment categories described by Law, McColl, and Stewart (1993). A biomechanical approach (from the physical rehabilitative category) will assist in gathering information and understanding how the work demands, the physical environment, and the workers' physical capabilities contribute to injuries that limit occupational performance. Similarly, use of organizational development approaches, from the environmental models category, will help in deciding what information to collect. These approaches will also guide the interpretation of the findings; in particular, how the organization of the work environment creates conditions that lead to injuries that hinder occupational performance. Collectively, they will be helpful in answering the question: What factors (personal or environmental) are contributing to workers' injuries?

Stage 3: Identify Occupational Performance Components and Environmental Conditions

The therapist uses a variety of assessment methods to gather needed information as noted in the contract. Objective observation and documentation of the job demands and work processes through direct observation and videotaping, a risk factors checklist, a retrospective injury record review, and review of work schedules are examples of assessments used to analyze the work site hazards. Analysis of the findings indicates that the occupational performance components and environmental conditions contributing to the occupational performance issue include

- Workers' physical fitness is less than is required for the job.
- Lack of knowledge of lifting techniques that can reduce risk of injury.
- The methods workers use to cope with the fast pace of work contribute to the higher risk of injury. For example, use of shortcuts such as lack of use of the recommended freezer protection clothing, and workers do not take the breaks that are requested by the employer.
- The physical and organizational work environment increases the risks of injury. For example, workers are rewarded for the amount of work completed rather than using safe work practices, work routines and schedules do not provide for variety in the physical demands of the work tasks, and workers indicate that there are not sufficient workers available during peak periods to carry out tasks in a timely manner and meet customers' needs.

Staff cutbacks due to downsizing occurred 6 months ago; the rate of injuries has increased since then. Workers initially used the shortcuts described as coping methods during the peak periods, but their use has recently become more frequent.

Stage 4: Identify Strengths and Resources

The managers of the plant and workers in the shipping and receiving departments have many strengths and resources that will be helpful in preventing worker injuries.

- Workers are committed to completing work requirements and ensuring customers are satisfied. Although this is a strength, it is also a limitation because workers complete their work even when it means working overtime, not taking breaks, and taking some shortcuts in recommended procedures.
- Staff turnover is low, and workers are very supportive of each other. They often help out in other work areas of the department when there is a lull in work in their own area.
- Managers and workers are eager to take the actions that are needed to reduce the risk of future injuries. They are enthusiastic about this even though they know this will necessitate some changes in work practices.
- All managers (in head office and the department) are readily accessible to workers and listen actively to their concerns.

- The company has allocated funds to develop and implement plans to prevent future injuries.
- The therapist has expertise in working with clients to solve problems that contribute to injuries in industrial settings. This expertise is recognized by the managers and workers.

Stage 5: Negotiate Targeted Outcomes and Develop Action Plans

Using the information that was collected in stages 1 and 3, a manager, the department heads, two worker representatives, and the occupational therapist work together to identify the goals they want to work toward and how they will reach them. This planning team decides on the targeted outcome(s) as well as the short-term objectives that will enable the targeted outcome to be achieved. Their plan includes the target dates for reaching the objectives and outcomes. At a meeting with other managers and workers, the proposed targeted outcomes, objectives, and plans are discussed and confirmed. Each person's role is identified and incorporated into the plan. Given the emphasis on eliminating injuries, a health promotion theoretical approach is added to those identified in stage 2.

Table 5-6 shows the targeted outcome. The pre-requisites to achieving the targeted outcome are

- Within 3 months, workers' physical fitness levels will be higher than prior to participation in the fitness program and will meet the minimum fitness level required for work.
- Within 1 month, workers will be able use safe lifting techniques correctly in all lifting.
- Within 3 months, work schedules and routines will vary the physical work requirements during shifts.
- Within 6 months, managers and department heads and workers will feel safe work is recognized and valued by the company; be satisfied with work schedules and routines; and report that the issue is resolved.

The following action plans are developed to achieve the short-term objectives that will lead to the targeted outcomes.

- The company will contract a fitness expert to provide a short-term supervised fitness program for workers. The occupational therapist will provide information to the fitness expert about the needs of the workers. The fitness expert will teach the workers how to lead such programs so that they can provide a lunchtime fitness program themselves that will help to maintain workers' fitness and health once the fitness expert's short-term contract ends.
- The therapist, in consultation with others, will develop and offer a back education program that will ensure that workers have the knowledge and skill needed to monitor their use of sound body mechanics and joint protection techniques when lifting. They will also be able to use this knowledge in educating new employees.

Table 5-6
Example 4: Client issues, components, environmental conditions, targeted outcomes, outcomes

Stage 1: Client identified OP problem and Stage 3: components and environmental conditions	Stage 5: Client targeted outcomes	Stage 7: Evaluate occupational performance outcomes
Potential for new injuries and/or recurring injuries among workers in the Shipping and Receiving Department related to:	Within six months of the completion of the occupational therapy program, no new or recurring injuries will have occurred among workers in the Shipping and Receiving Department.	With the exception of one injury that occurred because of inattention, no new or recurring injuries had occurred six months after the plans were implemented. The results suggest that the actions taken minimize the risk of injuries.
• Workers' physical fitness is less than is required for the job.		
• Lack of knowledge of lifting techniques that can reduce risk of injury.		
• Methods workers' use to cope with the fast pace of work contributes to the higher risk of injury.		
• The physical and organizational work environment increases the risks of injury.		

- The company will re-evaluate the personnel requirements in the shipping and receiving departments and, if needed, will hire more part-time workers to make safe work possible in regular and peak periods.
- The company, department heads, and workers, in consultation with the therapist, will develop and implement new work schedules and routines that facilitate the long-term maintenance of workers' fitness and health. They will also develop and implement a program that recognizes workers who work safely.

The occupational therapist has now completed all tasks specified in the contract that were negotiated in stage 1. Given the level of satisfaction with occupational therapy services to this point, the company, in consultation with the workers, extends the occupational therapy contract to implement the plans and evaluate the occupational performance outcomes.

Stage 6: Implement Plans Through Occupation

The plans are implemented as agreed. Although the plans identify the people who assume major roles in carrying out the plans, the company managers, the department heads, and the workers all participate. This enhances the likelihood that the outcomes will be achieved and maintained, because through active participation, all members of the company are contributing to the success (or failure) of the plan. The plans are more real and more meaningful. For example, workers' participation in the development of the variable workload routines increases their awareness of the challenges this brings for the company managers and department heads. Similarly, the re-evaluation of workloads and the demands for work increase the company managers' appreciation of the workload stresses the workers face.

Throughout implementation, the therapist coordinates the varied plans, monitors progress toward the targeted outcomes, and makes adjustments where they are necessary. The therapist assumes the role of coach. In this way, the company and all employees further develop their problem-solving skills so that they can apply them to future problems.

Stage 7: Evaluate Occupational Performance Outcomes

The targeted outcome for the occupational performance issue is noted in Table 5-6. Analysis of the findings for the short-term outcomes that were necessary to achieve the targeted outcome showed that

- the company had hired additional employees to assist during peak periods
- new work schedules and routines varied the physical work demands during shifts

Workers reported less stress and worry about injuries, that the company recognized and supported safety on the job, 85% of the workers met the minimum fitness level, 90% of workers attended the lunchtime fitness program regularly, workers used correct safe lifting techniques.

From a business perspective, other benefits were also evident. Workers' productivity had improved (i.e., more deliveries were made in the same time span and were on time, there were fewer order errors than prior to the program, and damage to goods was rare). Customers were also much more satisfied with the service.

The company managers and employees are very satisfied with the results and are committed to maintaining the changes that were introduced. They expect to have to make more changes in the future as work demands, technology, and equipment change. In this regard, they wish to contract the occupational therapy service on retainer, to ensure that they can be proactive rather than reactive in addressing future occupational performance issues.

This example shows that the Occupational Performance Process Model can be applied successfully with an organization. It can be done in many ways. In this instance, the process was divided into two parts with subsequent contracts negotiated as outcomes were met. The participation of management staff and workers, jointly and concurrently in all stages, demonstrated the positive outcomes of this client-centred approach. Because every organization has different needs, adjustments can be made in the number of contracts used to complete the process and the timing and sequence in which occupational performance issues are addressed. Stepping out of traditional service environments by offering services in the client's environment can be more meaningful for clients and more client-centred and also offer new exciting challenges for occupational therapists.

DISCUSSION

Occupational therapists who are firmly grounded in the principles, values, and client-centred process of their profession build bridges rather than barriers. They bring theory alive in practice through the behaviours they choose to exhibit, and they nurture the responding client behaviours that lead to healthy resolution of issues. They are focused on enabling occupation to the extent that barriers, such as institutional walls, lack of social policy, and bureaucracy, become challenges to be bridged rather than endpoints on a journey. These therapists can embrace change because their grounding is not in a specific location, or technique, or habit, but rather within themselves. These therapists provide leadership because they choose to and because there is really no other alternative if bridges are to be built. Using a client-centred occupational therapy process enables clients' occupations, and therapists' as well.

REFERENCES

Canadian Association of Occupational Therapists. (1996). Profile of occupational therapy practice in Canada. *Canadian Journal of Occupational Therapy, 63,* 79-95.

Fearing, V., Law, M., & Clark, J. (1997). An occupational performance process model: Fostering client and therapist alliances. *Canadian Journal of Occupational Therapy, 64,* 7-15.

Hobson, S. (1996). Reflections on: Being client-centred when the client is cognitively impaired. *Canadian Journal of Occupational Therapy, 63,* 133-137.

Law, M., Baptiste, S., Carswell, A., McColl, M., Polatajko, H., & Pollock, N. (1994). *The Canadian Occupational Performance Measure* (2nd ed.). Toronto, ON: CAOT Publications ACE.

Law, M., Cooper, B., Strong, S., Stewart, D., Rigby, P., & Letts, L. (1996). The person-environment-occupation model: A transactive approach to occupational performance. *Canadian Journal of Occupational Therapy, 63,* 9-23.

Mattingly, C. (1991). The narrative nature of clinical reasoning. *American Journal of Occupational Therapy, 45,* 998-1005.

McColl, M., Law, M., & Stewart, D. (1993). *Theoretical basis of occupational therapy: An annotated bibliography of applied theory in the professional literature.* Thorofare, NJ: SLACK Incorporated.

chapter

6

ASSESSMENT IN CLIENT-CENTRED OCCUPATIONAL THERAPY

NANCY POLLOCK, MSc, OT(C), MARY ANN McCOLL, PhD, OT(C)

Try to remember an instance recently when you were a client. Perhaps you bought a new computer, joined a fitness club, or had your car repaired. Now, try to remember the first interaction between yourself and the person who helped or served you. Did you feel that he or she understood what you wanted? Did you feel that he or she could offer you some expertise that would help you in getting what you wanted? Did you believe that you were ultimately going to get what you wanted? I use an example with which many of you will be able to identify.

I have a hairdresser who I have gone to faithfully for 15 years and have recommended to many friends and colleagues, and it's largely because of the relationship we have— a client-centred relationship. The first question that he always asks is, "What are we doing today?" Once I explain in everyday language what I'd like, he walks around, fingering my hair, tilting my head, presumably doing some kind of technical assessment about what will be required in order for me to have the haircut I want. He then lays out a plan of how we can achieve this hairdo—take a little off here, leave this part longer, and so on. I am often aware during this part of the interaction that he knows much more than he can tell me, but that he is disclosing fully enough for me to make a decision about whether or not to go ahead and start cutting. But it does not always go smoothly—sometimes there is an obstacle to the haircut I want. For example, it may be that my hair just won't do a certain thing. This is where the relationship is tested, and his true skill, both inter-personal and technical, is challenged. The challenge is to get me as close to the look I want as he can, while conforming to what my hair will do, all the while leaving me con-fident that he understands what I want and is going to help me to get it.

Although the context of a relationship with a therapist is considerably different from the relationship with a hairdresser or a computer salesperson, there are some interesting parallels that are pertinent to our discussion of client-centred occupational therapy.

This chapter is about assessment using a client-centred approach. Given that assess-ment often represents a therapist's first interaction with a client, it takes on enormous importance in establishing the nature of the relationship between a therapist and a client. Using a client-centred approach to assessment, clients tell therapists what their problems are; whereas using a traditional approach, therapists tell clients what their problems are.

The assessment offers therapists using a client-centred approach the opportunity to communicate to clients that they care about the client's view of the situation, that they want to understand the context of the person's life, that they are committed to helping, that they have some expertise that may be of assistance, and that they can be trusted to do what the client has said he or she wants.

This chapter will examine some of the assumptions of the client-centred approach and the implications of each for assessment. It will then analyze five different types of assessments used in occupational therapy, ranging from unstructured to structured, for suitability to the client-centred approach. Finally, the chapter will explore some issues raised in practice using client-centred assessment.

ASSESSMENT

Before proceeding, we must define three terms: assessment, client, and client-centred. The dictionary is of limited assistance in understanding what the term assessment means; it talks mostly about evaluating property and assessing taxes. Assessment is defined by Christiansen & Baum (1992) as "the process of gathering sufficient information about individuals and their environments to make informed decisions about intervention" (p. 376). The Canadian Association of Occupational Therapists (CAOT) (1991), in its national consensus guidelines for occupational therapy, defines assessment as "the process of collecting, analyzing and interpreting information, obtained through observation, interview, record review and testing" (p. 137). Either of these latter two definitions may serve our purposes in this chapter.

For our purposes, we will use the term assessment to refer to a two-tiered process: problem identification and problem analysis. At the first level, therapists, regardless of their therapeutic approach, must identify the problems that will be addressed in therapy. As occupational therapists, we are primarily interested in those problems for which we are qualified to assist; that is, problems of occupation. Problems are defined as those areas of occupation where clients indicate that they would like to pursue a change through therapy.

At the second level, therapists use further assessment techniques to analyze the problems identified: to understand why the problem exists, what causes it, what it feels like, how it is experienced by the client, what its history is, the context or environment in which the problem exists, and the consequences of the problem. Some examples of problems in occupational performance that might be identified at the first level are not being able to use public transportation, being unable to get in and out of the bathtub, not getting along with co-workers, being unable to care for one's child, or lacking opportunities to socialize. For any of these problems, the therapist must discover what is at the root of this problem and how can it best be addressed in therapy. Thus, the second level of assessment involves clinical reasoning, application of theory about occupation, and knowledge about humans and their environments. (See Chapter 4 for further discussion.)

CLIENT

The second term we must define for the purposes of our discussion of client-centred assessment is the term "client." Here, the dictionary is helpful; it defines a client as someone seeking the advice of a professional. The CAOT (1997) defines clients as "individuals with occupational problems arising from medical conditions, transitional difficulties, or environmental barriers. Clients may be organizations that influence occupational performance of particular groups or populations" (p. 180).

In the therapeutic context, we would add a further idea to the definition—that a client is someone who wishes to make a change through a process of therapy. In most instances, our clients will be people with disabilities who wish to solve problems relating to their occupational performance, with the assistance of an occupational therapist. However, this will not always be exclusively true. In some instances, individuals with disabilities may not be the ones in whom we expect to see change. For example, if we were working with a couple, one of whom had Alzheimer's Disease, we may not seek to make changes in the way the ill spouse functioned, but rather in the way the well spouse functioned. Thus, the well spouse is actually our client, although the name on the referral may be that of the ill spouse. Using another example, if we had a client with a disability who was having difficulties obtaining the appropriate accommodations in the workplace, we might consider the workplace, consisting of the physical environment, the co-workers, and management, our primary client, because they would be the locus of our efforts to facilitate change. This is an important idea to be clear about when discussing client-centred assessment, because if we are to assess our client, that is the person or environment in whom we seek to facilitate change, we must accurately identify the client and choose assessments that are appropriate to him, her, or it (the environment).

CLIENT-CENTRED

Our final definition refers to the term "client-centred." The words "client-centred" before the words "occupational therapy" refer to a way of practising occupational therapy (McColl, Gerein, & Valentine, 1997). They suggest a therapeutic orientation on the part of the therapist that not only places the wishes and issues of the client first, but in fact sees them as the only ones that are important. According to the client-centred approach, clients seek the assistance and support of a therapist to help them achieve their goals; and therapists provide an environment of understanding, trust, and acceptance that allows people to pursue changes toward their goals (Burnard & Morrison, 1991.)

By its very name, client-centred therapy differentiates itself from traditional biomedical approaches to therapy by calling the recipients of service clients. Unlike a patient, who is simply the object of service, a client seeks the advice of a professional in managing some aspect of his or her life (Herzberg, 1990; Patterson & Marks, 1992). Thus, the language implies that in a client-centred model, the client is in charge and is seeking from the relationship with the professional what he or she needs, and discarding that which he or she does not feel is necessary at this time.

As described in Chapter 1, the origins of client-centred practice are found in the work of Carl Rogers (1942). Rogers described client-centred therapy as a nondirective approach to therapy, where the therapist's role is to create an environment of trust and support, furnishing clients with the opportunity to utilize their own problem-solving capacities to realize their therapeutic goals. The client-centred approach has achieved considerable prominence in the past several years, yet the rhetoric associated with it often violates some of its fundamental assumptions. For example, we often hear about therapists "allowing clients to make decisions" or "involving clients in the process of therapy." Kerfoot and Leclair (1991) suggest that therapists may even use client-centred rhetoric as a means of guiding or manipulating the therapeutic agenda. Client-centred practice is not simply a more respectful way to deliver a professionally dominated or biomedical rehabilitation. Rather, it is a different model of service delivery altogether, where the therapist is engaged by the individual to assist with the achievement of personal goals in occupational performance.

ASSUMPTIONS OF THE CLIENT-CENTRED APPROACH

As client-centred occupational therapy has been described in this book, there are a number of assumptions that may assist us in understanding its implications for assessment (McColl, Gerein, & Valentine, 1997). The first assumption is that clients know what they want from therapy and what they need to reach their optimum level of occupational performance. Thus, the agenda for therapy is established by the client. This assumption is the ultimate extension of one of the most basic values of occupational therapists: the belief in the uniqueness and worth of every individual (Clarke, Scott, & Krupa, 1993). Further, this assumption allows therapists to trust clients to identify the problems that are most important to them and, thus, most important for therapy. In other words, for therapists who function from a client-centred perspective, there is no question of conflict between the problems that the therapist identifies and those that the client identifies, because the therapist understands his or her job in assessment as uncovering the problems for which the client is seeking help.

In some cases, clients may not be able to enumerate their problems clearly and succinctly in terms of occupational performance. They will almost certainly not use the language that therapists use to describe problems. For example, a client may say, "The mornings are such a hard time for me." In terms of occupational performance, this could mean

- My pain is very disabling first thing in the morning.
- My morning routine takes too long and I feel rushed.
- There are too many family demands on me when everyone is getting ready for work or school.
- By the time I get dressed, I have no energy left for anything else.
- I don't sleep well and feel groggy and irritable in the morning.
- My mood is very low at the start of the day.

The skill of the client-centred therapist in assessment lies in his or her ability to hear what people are saying they have difficulty with or are troubled by, and to understand their words in terms of problems of occupational performance.

People seeking occupational therapy may not be able to identify any problems initially; they may be motivated to seek therapy by a general sense of unease or discomfort with daily life and occupational roles. In those instances, the truly skilled client-centred therapist does not simply abandon the client-centred approach for a more professionally dominated approach. Instead, the therapist understands that there may be a therapeutic process associated with the ability of the client to identify problems. The therapist uses his or her expertise and understanding of occupational performance and health to assist clients to break down that feeling of unease according to frameworks that help occupational therapists understand problems. For example, they may attempt to break the problem down according to how it expresses itself in the domains of self-care, productivity, and leisure; they may attempt to ascertain whether the problem is experienced as a physical problem, an emotional problem, or a social problem; they may seek to understand whether the client sees the problem as existing within himself or herself or within the environment. All the while, therapist and client are moving toward a fuller and more detailed understanding of the problems that bring the client to therapy. But this is not all that is happening. The therapist is also communicating to the client an interest in understanding what the client wants from therapy, patience for the process, understanding of the uniqueness of the client's problems, and commitment to working through them together.

A second assumption of the client-centred approach is that the only relevant frame of reference or vantage point for therapy is that of the client. While the therapist may have knowledge and expertise about certain aspects of disability and therapy, he or she can never fully understand the values, beliefs, and experiences of the client and must, therefore, accept the client's reports as the most relevant source of information. This assumption is consistent with our understanding of occupation and disability, not as objective phenomena that can be observed and measured, but rather as subjective phenomena that must be understood from the perspective of the person experiencing them. For the first level of assessment, this assumption requires virtually all assessment within a client-centred approach to be self-report. Furthermore, it suggests that the more open-ended the assessment is, the greater the opportunity to hear the clients unedited, uncensored experience of occupation or disability. Thus open-ended assessments may produce richer, more accurate information about these subjective phenomena than more structured checklists, inventories, or indicators.

The third and final assumption affecting assessment and intervention is that the therapist cannot actually promote change; he or she can only create an environment that facilitates change. Change or new learning takes place only when an individual identifies it as necessary for the maintenance or development of the self (Rogers, 1965). Thus, any contention by the therapist that he or she is the agent of change is misguided, because the only agent of change can be the client him or herself. The most valuable role for the therapist is to support the client through the change with information, ideas, suggestions, and resources and to communicate to the client trust and belief in his or her ability to succeed in making the desired change.

The implication of this assumption for assessment is slightly more oblique, but it has to do with the nature of the therapeutic relationship and the extent to which this is largely established during the assessment. To the extent that a therapist maintains a client-centred approach throughout the process of assessment, a relationship may be established where a client understands that the therapist is not going to take over the process, is not going to assume sole responsibility for the success of therapy, and is not going to impose his or her will on the client. The dominance of professionals in the process of assessment and therapy has been shown to be, in fact, counter-therapeutic (Goodall, 1992). Professional dominance creates dependency, disempowerment, and, ultimately, institutionalization. Instead, a therapeutic relationship is established where the therapist shows belief in the potential of the client, enthusiasm about his or her ability to achieve goals and overcome problems, and knowledge and experience that may be marshaled to help.

ADVANTAGES AND DISADVANTAGES OF THE CLIENT-CENTRED APPROACH TO ASSESSMENT

The client-centred approach has a number of advantages and disadvantages over other approaches to assessment (McColl, Gerein, & Valentine, 1997). Its main advantage is its tendency to enhance the sense of mastery and control among clients (Emener, 1991; Goodall, 1992). This is accomplished in a number of ways: through communication of interest in the client's perceptions of his or her problems; through the therapist's commitment to assist the client with those problems; and through the therapist's communication of confidence in the client's ability to identify and solve problems.

A second advantage to the client-centred approach to assessment is the extent to which it supports a truly individualized or "tailored" approach to therapy (Brown, 1992). Because clients identify problems that are pertinent to their unique circumstances and context, occupational therapy interventions become explicitly framed in the context of that individual.

The third advantage of the client-centred approach is the opportunity that it presents for the therapist's own personal and professional growth and development. Unlike the traditional model, where the therapist is the expert and people are learning from him or her, in the client-centred model, the client is the expert. Thus, client-centred therapy provides an opportunity for the therapist to learn more about disability and its manifestations in people's lives, and more about the multidimensional nature of human occupation.

There are also a number of disadvantages to assessing from a client-centred perspective. Some clients appear to expect therapists to tell them what their problems are. For these clients, a therapist who will not take this role may be perceived as less skilled, less effective, or less cooperative (Schroeder & Bloom, 1979; Jaffe & Kipper, 1982; Wanigaratne & Barker, 1995).

A second disadvantage of the client-centred approach is the need for more assessments that support this approach to practice. A number of reviews of the literature show that there are few occupational therapy assessments that are suitable for application in a client-centred practice (Pollock, 1993; Pollock, Baptiste, Law, McColl, Opzoomer, & Polatajko, 1990; Trombly, 1993). This chapter goes on to review several of those identified.

Finally, a third disadvantage of client-centred assessment is that it may not be acceptable to all therapists. Rogers (1965) admits that the success or failure of client-centred therapy is often a function of the therapist's personality and his or her respect for others and belief in their resourcefulness and adaptiveness. To determine your own orientation toward client-centredness, ask yourself whose view prevails when client and therapist disagree about whether or not a client's performance on a particular occupational skill is satisfactory.

APPLICATION TO PRACTICE

While most therapists espouse a belief in client-centred practice, there is evidence of a gap between beliefs and actions. Neistadt (1995) surveyed occupational therapists working in adult physical rehabilitation facilities across the United States to assess the degree to which therapists incorporated client priorities into their treatment. Of the 267 respondents, 99% reported that they routinely identified client priorities upon admission. In contrast, Northen, Rust, Nelson, and Watts (1995) found through observation of initial assessments, again in adult rehabilitation settings, only 37% of the therapists tried to elicit clients' concerns, and none of the therapists asked the clients to establish priorities of concern. The difference between therapists' self-report and actual practice seems significant.

In another area of practice, working with young children and their families, the literature is full of discussions of the difficulties in implementing family-centred service (Bailey, Buysse, Smith, & Elam, 1992; Filer & Mahoney, 1996; Winton, McWilliam, Harrison, Owens, & Bailey, 1992). Collaborating with families in assessment and the establishment of goals are central to family-centred service, but appear to be quite difficult to do. Bailey (1988) identified five types of barriers to effective family assessment, including conceptual, measurement, interventionist, institutional, and family. The focus of this section will be on measurement barriers. I want to use a client-centred assessment approach, but how do I do it?

Neistadt (1995), in the survey of therapists in adult rehabilitation settings, asked whether the respondents assessed client priorities, but also asked *how* they assessed priorities. Ninety-five percent of the respondents reported using informal interviews. Neistadt states that

> "to establish treatment plans that will be maximally effective, occupational therapists must help clients evaluate and articulate what occupations have the most meaning to them. While informal interview can contribute to that process, it is not sufficient to precisely identify client priorities for treatment." (p. 435)

There are more formal methods of assessing client priorities in the literature. The following section will discuss these different methods, their strengths and limitations, and the issues raised for the therapists and the clients.

ASSESSMENT METHODS

There are a number of different methods the occupational therapist can use to help the client identify occupational performance problems. In this section, several types of approaches to assessment are presented along a continuum from unstructured to more structured methods. This is not meant to be an exhaustive inventory of available methods, but rather an overview of different types of assessment that can be used in client-centred practice. It is also important to remember that these assessment methods focus on the first tier of the process, that is, problem identification.

INFORMAL INTERVIEWS

The method that seems to make the most intuitive sense in relationships where one is providing a service is to ask the consumer of the service "What can I do for you?" or "How can I help you?" The client can then go on to describe their needs and what they would like to get out of the relationship. These types of open-ended questions can form a part of the initial interview with a new client. This type of questioning can quickly help to set a relaxed tone in an initial assessment and send a message to the client that the therapist is here to listen to his or her concerns. Problems arise, however, as most consumers of occupational therapy services are not familiar with what an occupational therapist does and, therefore, cannot identify what the therapist could do for them. We are not able to use a "tell me where it hurts" type of question, as the domain of our practice is much more complex and, often is not well understood by our clients. Clients are not likely to come to you and say, "I have lost the meaning in my daily occupations" or "I am unable to fulfill my role as homemaker and mother." The therapist must be able to explain the nature of occupation and occupational therapy to the client in terms that are meaningful to him or her. Then, perhaps, some clients will be able to articulate how they perceive their occupational performance problems.

Many of our clients, however, will not be able to respond to open-ended interview questions no matter what the content of the questions. They may have a cognitive impairment that limits their insight and judgment, e.g., a child with an intellectual handicap. They may have difficulty in communication, e.g., a person with aphasia. Other clients may be unsure of their occupational needs, e.g., a person who has recently experienced a stroke and has not yet realized the full impact of the stroke on his or her daily occupations. They may be hospitalized and unable to anticipate the consequences of their illness when they try to return home or return to work. There are many reasons why an individual may not be able to articulate the priorities of concern. In these instances, it will be important to re-think whether the individual is truly the client or whether the parent, spouse, or caregiver will be the person making the change in therapy and, therefore, the client with whom the interview should take place. It may be, however, that the individual is the appropriate respondent, but the method of assessment will need to be altered. They may require a more structured approach.

NARRATIVE AND LIFE HISTORY

The use of narrative methods and life histories has recently received increased attention in the occupational therapy literature. Frank (1996) reviewed a variety of narrative methods including case history, life charts, life history, life story, hermeneutic case reconstruction, and therapeutic employment. These methods all provide ways for clients to tell their story. Clark and Larson (1993) emphasized the importance of the use of these methods in the assessment process.

"... of utmost concern to therapists would be evoking personal narratives from their [patients] that reveal the meaning the [patient] derives from particular occupation, how they chunk or enfold their occupations, and how their occupational patterns flowing through the stream of time fit into a framework of how they understand their lives." (p. 55)

While much of the current literature focuses on the use of narrative methods in research, there are applications to clinical practice. The client and the therapist must collaborate in the telling of the life story. While the client has the story, the therapist can help the client to tell or write the story through questioning and probing. The therapist and client must also collaborate on the interpretation of the story, seeking meaning, reflecting themes, and identifying key events. It is this analysis of the story that differentiates the use of narrative methods from a more typical interview. For example, to help a client prepare for his or her first weekend home after a stroke, he or she and the therapist might collaborate to write a short story about leaving the hospital, driving home, arriving at the house, and entering the house with his or her now-altered physical capacity. Burke and Kern (1996) describe how narrative methods are typically interwoven in informal ways throughout the therapeutic interaction. They suggest that the use of these methods or the language describing these methods can help to inform the process of therapy and articulate client-centred issues.

METAPHOR

The use of metaphor can be a powerful therapeutic tool. Mallinson, Kielhofner, & Mattingly (1996) describe the use of metaphor as an alternative method to interpret narrative or life histories. While plot is often the focus of the telling of life stories, these authors suggest the search for metaphors or the search for what is implicit as well as explicit within the story can help both the client and the therapist bring meaning to the story. A metaphor, by definition, serves to represent something else, and may serve to simplify a complex story or reinforce recurring themes.

Metaphor can be used as a tool to interpret narrative passages or more explicitly as the passage itself. Hunt and Gow (1984) used the writing of a metaphor as a way to bring theoretical beliefs and frames of reference to the surface. Rochon (1994) used a similar exercise with occupational therapists to understand how they viewed practice. Similarly, it should be possible to engage some clients in writing metaphors to describe their experiences. Encouraging clients to complete phrases such as "For me, having a spinal cord injury is like ...." For example, a client might explain his or her experience through a metaphor like this:

"Living with schizophrenia makes me think of the mime character who moves as if he were trapped inside a glass box, always able to see the world around me, but never quite able to touch it, to experience it, or to be a part of it."

In another example, a client might compare the process of therapy to running a three-legged race with the therapist. This metaphor offers the opportunity to explore aspects of the process of therapy and how it appears to the client. The therapist might ask

- How did we pick each other as partners for the three-legged race?
- What is the scarf or band that is holding us together?
- How tight or loose is the band?
- How long is this race?
- What is at the end?
- With whom are we competing?
- Who is setting the pace?
- Does the way we run together change over the course of the race?

By discussing the content of the metaphor and the meaning it holds for the individual, a great deal can be learned about the client's life experience and perspective. Obviously, the use of metaphor with clients requires a degree of sophistication that not all clients will possess. These types of exercises may be very powerful for some and quite inappropriate for others.

SEMI-STRUCTURED INTERVIEW

Another method available to therapists is the use of more structured interviews. These provide the therapist with specific questions to guide the interview, or with areas on which to focus in seeking information from the client. Two examples of these more structured interviews from the occupational therapy literature include the Occupational Performance History Interview (OPHI) (Kielhofner & Henry, 1988) and the Canadian Occupational Performance Measure (COPM) (Law, Baptiste, Carswell, McColl, Polatajko, & Pollock, 1994). The OPHI consists of 39 recommended questions and covers five content areas: organization of daily routines, life roles, interests, values, and goals; perceptions of ability and responsibility; and environmental influences. The OPHI provides a structure to elicit the client's life history in that it focuses on the past and the present for each of the areas. There is also an accompanying Life History Narrative Form used to summarize qualitative findings from the interview. The OPHI is scored by the therapist on a five-point scale from 5=adaptive to 1=maladaptive. For example, within the area of organization of daily routines, a client with multiple sclerosis might describe the differences in a typical day before and after a recent exacerbation in the condition. By exploring these differences and the client's satisfaction with the present routine, areas for focus in therapy may become evident. The OPHI, like any interview, is dependent on the therapist's skill in conducting the interview and establishing rapport with the client. Because the therapist is the rater of adaptation, it is also influenced by the therapist's frame of reference. Reliability studies have shown the instrument to be only moderately stable with a fair degree of variability between raters (Kielhofner & Henry, 1988; Kielhofner, Henry, Walens, & Rogers, 1991). The OPHI was found to be sensitive to change in a sample of people with spinal cord injury (Lynch & Bridle, 1993).

The COPM also provides a structure for the interview with the client, but focuses on the identification of problems in the areas of self-care, productivity, and leisure. Specific interview questions are not provided, but rather a framework is used to help the client articulate the difficulties he or she is encountering in his or her daily life. The scoring differs from the OPHI in that the client does the rating. A 1 to 10 scale is used for scoring identified occupational performance issues in the three domains. Once the client has identified the things he or she would like to be able to do, he or she rates the importance of those activities. This serves to establish the client's priorities and leads very naturally into intervention planning. The client then goes on to rate the most important items on his or her current performance and satisfaction with that performance. Again, in the client with multiple sclerosis mentioned above, her COPM results may look like this:

Problem	Importance	Performance	Satisfaction
Climbing stairs	10	2	1
Preparing meals	10	4	3
Child care	10	1	1
House cleaning	8	3	5
Reading	7	5	2

The COPM interview highlights the priority concerns from the client's perspective and provides a baseline assessment for measuring outcomes on reassessment. The COPM has been used with a broad spectrum of clients and has been shown to have good to excellent test-retest reliability, to be very responsive to change after occupational therapy intervention, and to correlate highly with measures of similar constructs (Law, Baptiste, Carswell, McColl, Polatajko, & Pollock, 1994).

In an effort to focus outcome measurement toward functional outcomes of significance to the client, some authors have developed more individualized measures. This has been driven by the move to the provision of client-centred service as well as the need to find outcome measures that are more responsive to change and, hence, able to detect clinically and statistically significant differences between experimental and control groups in randomized trials. An example, found outside the occupational therapy literature, of a measure more responsive to individual differences is the MACTAR Patient Preference Disability Questionnaire (Tugwell, Bombardier, Buchanan, Goldsmith, Grace, & Hanna,

1987). Although described as a questionnaire, the MACTAR is in the form of an interview. It has been designed for clients with arthritis, although could easily be modified for clients experiencing other types of illness or disability. The client is asked to identify the daily activities that are affected by the arthritis. Some prompt questions are listed to ensure the client thinks about all the different types of daily activities including work, recreation, household management, and social activities. The client is then asked to rank the activities in order of importance, that is, which of these activities would you most like to be able to do without the pain or discomfort of your arthritis (Tugwell, Bombardier, Buchanan, Goldsmith, Grace, & Hanna, 1987). Using a Problem Elicitation Technique (PET), the client then goes on to identify the level of difficulty experienced in each task (Buchbinder, Bombardier, Yeung, & Tugwell, 1995). These ratings are multiplied by the importance ratings resulting in a total score. This methodology is very similar to the one used in the COPM.

This type of assessment approach can help to focus the therapy on the issues most important to the client and make the problem identification process more relevant. As noted by Buchbinder, Bombardier, Yeung, & Tugwell (1995), "... many items identified as important by the patient do not appear on conventional questionnaires, and even the most frequently identified disabilities are either not mentioned at all or classified as unimportant by many other patients" (p. 1569).

This type of PET technique could be adapted for use with many different types of clients by simply removing the word arthritis from the initial prompt question and inserting whatever the illness/injury/disability may be in the case of the client being interviewed.

HEALTH AND FUNCTIONAL STATUS QUESTIONNAIRES

There are a multitude of health status and functional status questionnaires in the health care literature. These measures are designed to tap a wide range of health status states or levels of functional limitations. They are designed to be inclusive and comprehensive, may be based on self-report or interview, and measure the full range of health from well-being to disability. An example of a global health status measure is the SF-36, arising from the Medical Outcomes Study (Ware & Sherbourne, 1992). In contrast to many health surveys that are diagnosis- or age-specific, the SF-36 was designed for use with a wide variety of clients. It includes 36 items that tap eight health concepts: physical functioning, role limitations because of physical health problems, bodily pain, social functioning, general mental health, role limitations because of emotional problems, vitality, and general health perceptions. While the SF-36 covers a wide breadth of health indicators, it is limited in its depth, e.g., there is only one question focusing on daily self-care activities. It can serve to provide an overview from the client's perspective, but would need to be supplemented by additional assessment in most cases.

The Functional Status Questionnaire (FSQ) (Jette & Cleary, 1986) is another example of a global status measure. It includes the domains of physical function, psychological function, and social-role function. A series of questions guide the client through a review of the activities of the past month and determine the degree of impact of the illness/injury/disability on function. Unlike most of the methods described in this chapter, the FSQ is a normed measure and suggests whether clients are scoring in an "acceptable range" or in a "warning zone." While the FSQ covers important areas of functional impact, the fact that the scoring system was developed by a consensus panel suggests it has limited value as a client-centred measure. The importance to the client of the different areas of function are not considered. In a review of five health status measures, McHorney and Tarlov (1995) concluded that the measures lacked precision and were of limited usefulness in individual client assessment.

ISSUES ARISING IN CLIENT-CENTRED ASSESSMENT

The essence of a therapeutic interaction being client-centred demands that it be tailored to the needs of the client. This requires the therapist to respond and adapt to an infinite array of communication styles, preferences, levels of structure required, contexts, and issues. This chapter has presented some different methods of conducting the initial assessment, but the real skill lies in choosing the method that best fits the client and in conducting the assessment in an effective manner. As Frank (1996) states in describing the various life history approaches "... what really matters is that the work of understanding patients' lives is done well" (p. 252). The rest of your relationship with the client, the goals that are set, the direction of the intervention, the measurement of the outcomes, and the decisions on when to terminate the relationship all flow from this initial client assessment.

Three issues that frequently come up in discussions of the use of client-centred assessment methods are time, client insight, and contextual fit. Occupational therapists frequently state that they don't have time for these types of assessments. They may only have one opportunity to see the client, or they may have restricted time for the initial interview. Therapists may feel these methods are an add-on to their already busy assessment schedule. That is likely because the therapist is considering only the second tier of the assessment process: the analysis of factors causing the occupational performance problem. As occupational therapists, our domain of concern is occupation, a personal, contextual construct. We must understand the nature of the client's occupation before we can move on to any meaningful intervention. The use of methods to identify the occupational issues from the client's perspective should, in fact, save time, as they serve to focus the plan on areas meaningful to the client and actively engage them in the therapeutic process from the outset. These methods free the therapist from more "comprehensive" or time-consuming assessment batteries that gather a great deal of data, but hold little relevance for the client. How often do we describe clients as noncompliant without examining whether the intervention has any meaning for the individual? For example, a therapist working in the community is seeing a client with rheumatoid arthritis for the first time. The therapist routinely does a physical assessment and an activities of daily living assessment on her first visit. In this case, the client's concerns actually centre on accessing the community and how to effectively negotiate transportation. She is very satisfied with how she is managing her self-care, and the family has worked out a good system of support. For the client and the therapist, this assessment will have been a waste of time and will not lead to dealing with the issues of concern. If the visit had started with an interview or assessment, such as the COPM or MACTAR, considerable time would have been saved.

A second issue frequently raised is client insight. All of the methods of client-centred assessment described here rely on the clients to respond to questions and examine and articulate their occupational performance issues. For some, this will be difficult, if not impossible. In these instances it is important to consider again the question "who is the client?" It may be that it is broader than the individual named on the referral. It may be the spouse, the parent, the family, the professional caregiver, the workplace, etc. Those close to the client may serve as the respondents in the assessment. It is important, however, to distinguish between these individuals as proxies for the client and as the clients themselves. For example, the husband of a woman with Alzheimer's disease cannot answer questions about what is important for his wife. He must answer about what is important for him in caring for and perhaps living with his wife. He is the client in this situation. He is the one who is seeking to make changes. Similarly, young children may not have developed the ability to assess their own situations or may not be concerned about environmental expectations. A child with Attention Deficit Disorder may not be concerned about his or her disruptive behaviour, but for the teacher, it is the key issue and must be dealt with before the teacher will engage in any carry over of therapy to the classroom.

It is also important not to make assumptions about a client's level of insight. Therapists have been surprised on more than a few occasions by the ability of a client, previously thought to be incompetent, to articulate his or her needs. Where possible, seek the client's input and then include those around the client.

A third issue to consider is context. Client-centred therapy is difficult to practice in a system dominated and structured by a biomedical model. The therapist needs to examine the values that guide his or her practice and look at the system within which he or she is working. Pragmatic issues such as team philosophies, charting and reporting requirements, limitations on visits allowed, etc., can make it very challenging for the therapist striving to practice in a client-centred manner. It is important to analyze these factors and be aware of obstacles that may exist in the current system. Awareness of the "fit" of the practice model can go a long way toward overcoming barriers. For example, an occupational therapist practising on a burn unit in an acute-care hospital may have a very specific role targeted at symptom relief and prevention, perhaps through the use of splinting and pressure garments. At this early stage post-injury, consideration of the client's perspective on his or her occupational performance is not central to the therapy process. Care can still be delivered in a respectful manner, but it is unlikely to be truly client-centred.

SUMMARY

The initial assessment often represents the first interaction between clients and therapists and, therefore, takes on tremendous importance. The assessment process sends a strong message about the nature of the relationship between client and therapist. For those using a client-centred approach, the initial step in assessment is to hear what the client's concerns are and what he or she would like to get out of therapy. In this approach, clients' wishes and issues are paramount. The agenda is established by the client. For some clients, this will be easy to do, and the therapist need only listen. For some clients, however, the recognition or identification of occupational problems is extremely difficult. It is here where the therapist's skills are truly challenged.

This chapter has presented several different methods of engaging the client in identifying his or her priorities and concerns. Each has its own strengths and limitations. The important issue is that the therapist enable the client to articulate the occupational performance issues that he or she is faced with. Therapists must use their skills to select the appropriate method for the particular client and adapt it to the situation. It is not easy. It requires flexibility, interpersonal skill, active listening, empathy, and patience. These methods of assessment often represent a shift in thinking for the therapist, a move away from the way they may have been trained, and some discomfort as they move toward a new type of relationship with clients. It may be more comfortable to use a standardized measure to assess a performance component than it is to open the discussion to whatever the client may want to deal with. But, it is essential to establishing a client-centred relationship and will guide the rest of the therapeutic process.

REFERENCES

Bailey, D. B. (1988). Rationale and model for family assessment in early intervention. In D. B. Bailey & R. J. Simeonsson (Eds.). *Family assessment in early intervention*. Columbus, OH: Merrill Publishing.

Bailey, D. B., Buysse, V., Smith, T., & Elam, J. (1992). The effects and perceptions of family involvement in program decisions about family-centered practices. *Evaluation and Program Planning, 15,* 23-32.

Brown, S. J. (1992). Tailoring nursing care to the individual client: Empirical challenge of a theoretical concept. *Research in Nursing and Health, 15,* 39-46.

Buchbinder, R., Bombardier, C., Yeung, M., & Tugwell, P. (1995). Which outcome measures should be used in rheumatoid arthritis clinical trials? *Arthritis & Rheumatism, 38,* 1568-1580.

Burke, J. P., & Kern, S. B. (1996). Is the use of life history and narrative in clinical practice reimbursable? Is it occupational therapy? *American Journal of Occupational Therapy, 50,* 389-392.

Burnard, P., & Morrison, P. (1991). Client-centred counselling: A study of nurses' attitudes. *Nurse Education Today, 11,* 104-109.

Canadian Association of Occupational Therapists (1991). *Occupational therapy guidelines for client-centred practice.* Toronto, ON: Author.

Canadian Association of Occupational Therapists (1997). *Enabling occupation: A Canadian occupational therapy perspective* (Draft). Ottawa, ON: Author.

Christiansen, C., & Baum, C. (1992). *Occupational therapy: Overcoming human performance deficits.* Thorofare, NJ: SLACK Incorporated.

Clark, F., & Larson, E. (1993). Developing an academic discipline: The science of occupation. In H. Hopkins & H. Smith (Eds.). *Willard and Spackman's occupational therapy* (8th ed.). Philadelphia: Lippincott, pp. 44-57.

Clarke, C., Scott, E., & Krupa, T. (1993). Involving clients in program evaluation and research. *Canadian Journal of Occupational Therapy, 60,* 192-199.

Emener, W. G. (1991). Empowerment in rehabilitation: An empowerment philosophy for rehabilitation in the 20th century. *Journal of Rehabilitation, 57*(4), 7-12.

Filer, J. D., & Mahoney, G. J. (1996). Collaboration between families and early intervention service providers. *Infants and Young Children, 9,* 22-30.

Frank, G. (1996). Life histories in occupational therapy clinical practice. *American Journal of Occupational Therapy, 50,* 251-264.

Goodall, C. (1992). Preserving dignity for disabled people. *Nursing Standard, 6*(35), 25-27.

Herzberg, S. R. (1990). Client or patient: Which term is more appropriate for use in occupational therapy? *American Journal of Occupational Therapy, 44,* 561-565.

Hunt, D. E., & Gow, J. (1984). How to be your own best theorist II. *Theory into Practice, 18,* 64-71.

Jaffe, Y., & Kipper, D. A. (1982). Appeal of rational-emotive and client-centred therapies to first-year psychology and non-psychology students. *Psychological Reports, 50,* 781-782.

Jette, A. M., & Cleary, P. D. (1986). Functional disability assessment. *Physical Therapy, 67,* 1854-1859.

Kerfoot, K. M., & Leclair, C. (1991). Building a patient-focused unit: The nurse manager's challenge. *Nursing Economics, 9,* 441-443.

Kielhofner, G., & Henry, A. D. (1988). Development and investigation of the Occupational Performance History Interview. *American Journal of Occupational Therapy, 42,* 489-498.

Kielhofner, G., Henry, A. D., Walens, D., & Rogers, E. S. (1991). A generalizability study of the Occupational Performance History Interview. *The Occupational Therapy Journal of Research, 11,* 292-306.

Law, M., Baptiste, S., Carswell, A., McColl, M. A., Polatajko, H., & Pollock, N. (1994). *The Canadian Occupational Performance Measure* (2nd ed.). Toronto, ON: CAOT Publications.

Lynch, K. B., & Bridle, M. J. (1993). Construct validity of the OPHI. *The Occupational Therapy Journal of Research, 13,* 231-240.

Mallinson, T., Kielhofner, G., & Mattingly, C. (1996). Metaphor and meaning in a clinical interview. *American Journal of Occupational Therapy, 50,* 338-346.

McColl, M. A., Gerein, N., & Valentine, F. (1997). Meeting the challenge of disability: Models for enabling function and well-being. In C. Christiansen & C. Baum (Eds.). *Occupational therapy: enabling function and well-being* (2nd ed.). Thorofare NJ: SLACK Incorporated, pp. 508-529.

McHorney, C. A., & Tarlov, A. R. (1995). Individual-patient monitoring in clinical practice: Are available health status surveys adequate? *Quality of Life Research, 4,* 293-307.

Neistadt, M. E. (1995). Methods of assessing clients' priorities: A survey of adult physical dysfunction settings. *American Journal of Occupational Therapy, 49,* 428-436.

Northen, J. G., Rust, D. M., Nelson, C. E., & Watts, J. H. (1995). Involvement of adult rehabilitation patients in setting occupational therapy goals. *American Journal of Occupational Therapy, 49,* 214-220.

Patterson, J. B., & Marks, C. (1992). The client as customer: Achieving service quality and customer satisfaction in rehabilitation. *Journal of Rehabilitation, 58*(4), 16-20.

Pollock, N. (1993). Client-centred assessment. *American Journal of Occupational Therapy, 47,* 298-301.

Pollock, N., Baptiste, S., Law, M., McColl, M. A., Opzoomer, A., & Polatajko, H. (1990). Occupational performance measures: A review based on the Guidelines for Client-centred Practice. *Canadian Journal of Occupational Therapy, 57,* 82-87.

Rochon, S. M. (1994). *Theory from practice: An effective curriculum for occupational therapists.* Unpublished master's thesis, McMaster University, Hamilton, Ontario, Canada.

Rogers, C. (1942). *Counselling and psychotherapy: Newer concepts in practice.* Boston: Houghton-Mifflin Co.

Rogers, C. (1965). *Client-centred therapy: Its current practice, implications and theory.* Boston: Houghton-Mifflin Co.

Schroeder, D. H., & Bloom, L. J. (1979). Attraction to therapy and therapist credibility as a function of therapy orientation. *Journal of Clinical Psychology, 35,* 683-686.

Trombly, C. (1993). Anticipating the future: Assessment of occupational function. *American Journal of Occupational Therapy, 47,* 253-257.

Tugwell, P., Bombardier, C., Buchanan, W. W., Goldsmith, C. H., Grace, E., & Hanna, B. (1987). The MACTAR Patient preference Disability Questionnaire—An individualized functional priority approach for assessing improvement in physical disability in clinical trials in rheumatoid arthritis. *Journal of Rheumatology, 14,* 446-451.

Wanigaratne, S., & Barker, C. (1995). Clients' preferences for styles of therapy. *British Journal of Clinical Psychology, 34,* 215-222.

Ware, J. E., & Sherbourne, C. D. (1992). The MOS 36-item short-form health survey (SF-36). 1. Conceptual framework and item selection. *Medical Care, 30*, 473-483.

Winton, P. J., McWilliam, P. J., Harrison, T., Owens, A. M., & Bailey, D. B. (1992). Lessons learned from implementing a team-based model for change. *Infants and Young Children, 5*, 49-57.

RESOURCES

Canadian Occupational Performance Measure
Canadian Association of Occupational Therapists
CTTC, Suite 3400
1125 Colonel By Drive
Ottawa, Ontario K1S 5R1

or

American Occupational Therapy Association
4720 Montgomery Lane
P.O. Box 31220
Bethesda, MD 20824-1220

A User's Guide to the Occupational Performance
History Interview
American Occupational Therapy Association
PO Box 31220
Bethesda, MD 20824-1220

SF-36
Medical Outcomes Trust
20 Park Plaza
Suite 1014
Boston, MA 02116-4313

Functional Status Index
Allen Jette
MGH Institute of Health Professions
15 River Street
Boston, MA 02108-3402

Engaging the Person in the Process: Planning together for Occupational Therapy Intervention

Leonard N. Matheson, PhD

In order for the occupational therapy process to be optimally effective, the client must be actively engaged in a process. In fact, the client is at the centre of the process that is facilitated by the therapist. Facilitation of the therapeutic process begins with an invitation and proceeds to initiation and engagement in subsequent therapeutic tasks, each of which must be engaged anew.

HISTORICAL UNDERPINNINGS

Engagement in therapy is basic to all therapeutic enterprises. The client-centred approach to engagement in occupational therapy borrows from the client-centred approach to psychotherapy developed by Carl Rogers (Kirschenbaum & Henderson, 1989; Rogers, 1961, 1980) as well as the work of Abraham Maslow (1968, 1971), Robert White (1959, 1971), Albert Bandura (1989, 1990), and Martin E. P. Seligman (1975, 1991).

Carl Rogers (1961) was the leading proponent of the client-centred approach to psychotherapy. He emphasized the need for the therapist to be genuinely involved in the therapeutic relationship on a personal basis, transcending the professional façade. He also stressed the need for the client to have "unconditional positive regard" from the therapist and that the therapist must develop an empathic understanding of the client.

Abraham Maslow (1968) studied people whom he described as "actualizing;" those people who were developing to the boundaries of their potential. For Maslow, therapy occurs, in part, by assisting the individual to become aware of his or her identity and how that can be expressed in the individual's occupational roles. People who are self-actualizing integrate their occupational roles as part of the self. A basic therapeutic task to facilitate actualization involves helping the client to uncover his or her goals and priorities so that they can be actively addressed.

Robert White (1959) made many important contributions to the concept of occupational competence and is a central theorist in the development of the "occupational competence model of human development" (Matheson & Bohr, 1997). Although he was not a therapist, he described adaptation as a consequence of the person's striving to achieve an acceptable compromise with the environment (White, 1974) in order to optimize occupational role function (Baum, 1991). He brought attention to the need for a view of the person as inherently motivated to become competent (White, 1971), which has had significant effect on the practice of occupational therapy.

Albert Bandura's work (1989, 1990) on the central importance of self-efficacy and personal agency in human development stresses the person's perceptions of abilities through the effect of this perception on how the person behaves and his or her level of motivation, thought processes, and emotional reactions to challenging circumstances. By extension, therapeutic effect begins with an understanding of the client's circumstance as viewed by the client.

Martin E. P. Seligman (1975, 1991) has made recent important contributions to the understanding of psychological health and motivation, which are based on the person's cognitive appraisal of his or her circumstances and the events that the person experiences. Integrating the psychotherapeutic approaches developed by Aaron T. Beck (1976) and Albert Ellis (1979), Seligman presents methods that can be used by occupational therapists to facilitate their clients' development of accurate and growth-enhancing self-communications.

All of these approaches to therapy are based on the establishment and maintenance of engagement. When engagement is done well, the client will be optimally motivated to pursue the goals of therapy. In addition, the client will be more likely to actively negotiate adjustment in goals as therapy unfolds, and collaborate in working with the therapist. Conversely, when engagement is not done well or is forced, casual, or taken for granted, the therapeutic dyad often is troubled, and therapeutic effect is limited.

PERTINENT CHARACTERISTICS OF THE PROCESS

Therapeutic engagement is purpose-driven. It is not casual, nor does it occur with spurious intent. It is not merely for the purpose of communicating with or knowing the client that the therapist is involved. It is based on the notions that the therapist can be helpful and that the client will find this to be true. This is the core of the purpose of all types of therapeutic engagement.

Therapeutic engagement is person-centred, a state that is more basic than client-centred, because being a person is more basic and encompassing than being a client, which is a temporary and relatively narrow role. The engagement process is personal and intimate, unique to the individual and to the therapeutic dyad composed of the person and his or her therapist. It relies on the availability of the person who is the therapist and requires that this person be emotionally healthy, secure, and possess those characteristics that are sought by the person who is the client. The personal nature of this engagement is true even when the client's caregiver or parent is also the therapist's client. In such circumstances, the interpersonal interactions can become as complex as those in other person-to-person relationships that occur in nontherapeutic life situations. A person-centred approach in this circumstance requires that individual relationships be established between the person who is the therapist and each person who is a client, recognising the relationship that each has with the other. A simple depiction of a two-member dyadic model is presented in Figure 7-1.

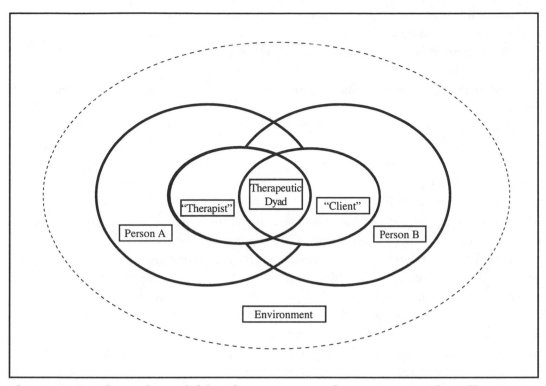

Figure 7-1. The roles within the persons who compose the client-centred therapeutic dyad.

Each person in the therapeutic dyad acts through his or her respective role of therapist or as client. To the degree that the person who is the therapist is able to interact with the person who is the client, the dyadic relationship will be genuine. Thus, the availability of the person who is the therapist is fundamental to engagement of the client in the process of client-centred occupational therapy.

The possibility of distinction between the goals found within the therapist's role and the goals of the person who is the therapist with unique values and beliefs is unique to the client-centred approach to therapy. It requires that the person who is the therapist be internally congruent. The therapist who is "performing" this role is going to be much less able to engage the person who is the client than the therapist who is "living" this role. For the effective client-centred therapist, this congruence leads to a natural blending of professional and personal goals. When this congruence is not present, it will be difficult for the therapist to be client-centred. Another way to say this is that the client-centred approach is not based on techniques, although techniques may be used by the client-centred therapist. For example, the therapist who experiences frustration with limitations experienced by the client will be more likely to report or display those frustrations to the client if he or she is involved in a client-centred therapeutic relationship because, to maintain consistency with one's self, reports or displays of those feelings is necessary. Such reports or displays have two immediate benefits: The first is that the client realizes that the therapist is understanding the client's circumstances. The second is reported by experienced therapists to be an increased awareness of those circumstances. Once reported to the client, these frustrations often become dissipated and will decrease in importance. It may be that therapists who do not report or display emotional consequences of clients' circumstances become emotionally blunted to those circumstances, losing awareness and sensitivity.

The client-centred approach must be based on a genuine interest in the person who is the client held by the person who is the professional. If the therapist is unable to step beyond his or her role and be available as a person, it is not reasonable to expect that the client will do the same. It is entirely possible that, with a particular client or at a particular point in a therapist's life, stepping beyond the therapist role to share with the person who is the client, the goals of the person who is the therapist will not be possible. When this is the case, an effective client-centred relationship will not occur. This can occur when the therapist is so different from the client that they do not share enough to be personally engaged, or in situations in which personal attributes of one are not acceptable to the other. It can also occur when the therapist is not professionally secure enough to step beyond the formal boundaries that guide "professional" participation and interaction. The word "professional" was placed in quotes in the prior sentence to indicate that formal policies and procedures exist for professionals that must be followed. This approach requires that these rules be a starting point and must not be violated, but will become the building blocks of a person-to-person relationship. Some therapists don't have the ability to step beyond these basics. Other therapists experience periods in their lives when temporary withdrawal to the confines of these rules is necessary due to circumstances that do not directly affect the therapeutic dyad, such as familial discord that is experienced by the therapist or disruptions of the therapist's health. During these periods, it may be necessary for the therapist to enter a therapeutic relationship as a client, seeking out a counselor who appreciates the demands that helping others entails.

Can there be confusion of goals, priorities, and conduct in the client-centred approach? Certainly, as there often is in other approaches. What is distinct about the client-centred approach stems from the nature of this confusion and its antidote: Confusion will occur when the therapeutic dyad strays from the values, goals, and abilities of the person who is the client. Are there limits to the values, goals, and abilities of the person who is the client? Certainly, there must always be limits that exist in the environment and that are manifest in the people and roles that compose the therapeutic dyad. The limits are usually rational, knowable, and known to the therapist, who contributes this information to the therapeutic dyad, which allows the dyad to develop in a healthy and environmentally congruent manner. The modeling of appropriate client-therapist behavior is the responsibility of the therapist, because the client is new to his or her role while the therapist is experienced in his or her role.

Therapeutic engagement is enabling of the development of the person who is the client. It is unencumbering of limitations, facilitative of growth, accommodating of the client's abilities and limitations, and affirming of his or her competence.

CHARACTERISTICS OF THE PERSON WHO IS THE CLIENT

The person who is the client has an innate urge toward competence (White, 1971) that provides the motivation for participating in occupational role activities. This also provides the motivation for participation in the occupational therapy process. The mechanism of the development of competence has been described elsewhere (Matheson & Bohr, 1997). Briefly, competence develops at the interface between the individual's effectancies, the role's challenges, and the environment's affordances. The first component of this triad—abilities—is defined as the immediate capacity of the person to respond. Effectancies are based on the abilities that the person has that are stimulated by his or her role challenges, which is the second component of the triad. For example, the ability of a child to throw a baseball will develop naturally from early childhood through adolescence. If the child becomes a member of a baseball team, the development of this ability will be stimulated because it is demanded by the "teammate" role. An ability that is stimulated by role demands is termed an effectancy. Effectancies have a more rapid development curve than abilities and are maintained at a higher level than abilities. To return to the above example, if the child takes on the role of pitcher on the team, the effectancy for throwing a baseball will develop at a different rate and to a different level and with different qualities than if the child is an outfielder. In each teammate role, however, it can be expected that the effectancy will differ from the ability in that the effectancy's level of performance will be higher. After the child reaches adulthood, if the effectancy becomes an ability because it is no longer stimulated by the role demands, the performance level will stagnate and gradually deteriorate as age changes occur. If it remains an effectancy because it is stimulated by role demands, it will remain at a higher level for a longer period in spite of age changes. Why is the distinction between abilities and affordances important? Because it is often forgotten that ability is dependent on demand posed by role challenges. Thus, using the term effectancy provides an emphasis or a reminder that important qualitative differences exist that are a result of active occupational involvement. Challenges come from the role and are those demands of the role that extend beyond the person's abilities (immediate capacity to respond) as the role is undertaken. Growth occurs as the person adapts to a role challenge. Growth occurs in the service of occupational competence, which is the driving force behind all occupational development. Stagnation and deterioration occur when the challenge is missing, whether due to role changes such as retirement or due to an impairment-producing injury. If disability is the inadequacy of ability, its remediation is the development of effectancies.

The third component of the triad is affordances, which are characteristics of the environment that are uniquely identified by the person based on his or her cognitive style, experience, and ability. Early use of environmental affordances to bridge the gap between role demands and personal resources allows the individual's effectancies to further develop. Competence is achieved when the role tasks are adequately performed through a combination of effectancies and affordances. Competence is maintained through a stable ongoing balance between effectancies and affordances that are adequate to meet occupational role challenges.

The therapeutic experience is unnatural, not normally a component of the development of the person. For most people, healthy development does not require a therapist. As a consequence, an additional characteristic of the person who is the client must be identified: his or her psychological availability for therapy. People have attitudes about therapy and therapists that can lead to resistance to or rejection of therapeutic involvement. To the degree that this is found in the individual client, it must be respected and addressed as the entry point for engagement. To the degree that the client is available, the therapeutic dyad can be vigorous and negotiative.

CHARACTERISTICS OF THE ENVIRONMENT

The client's environment contains aspects that are innocuous, threatening, accommodative, and supportive. The innocuous aspects of the environment are not perceived by the client or, if they are perceived and judged to be innocuous, are disregarded. Threatening aspects of the environment are perceived by the client and are judged to be an impediment to the completion of the tasks that comprise the occupational role. The environmental threats can frustrate, limit, or prevent the client from performing these tasks. Thus, in order to achieve competence, the client must deal with them. Accommodative aspects of the environment are those with which the client must be passively involved. The client perceives these aspects to be both nonthreatening and nonfacilitative. These aspects of the environment are neutral, but are not innocuous.

The occupational therapist is unique among health care professionals in that the focus of the occupational therapist's involvement is on this environmental aspect of the development of competence. For example, Peter Jones (a real person with a fictitious name) was 15 years old when he suffered a C5-6 spinal cord injury during a high school football game and became quadriplegic. Although Peter had all of the necessary medical care and rehabilitation, and received excellent support from his family and friends, he became depressed, withdrawn, and suicidal. From his point of view, the assistance he was offered was not pertinent to his goals of being a football player and high school student once again, and he had no other goals to pursue. Because Peter could not identify a role in which he might be able to demonstrate competence, he did not utilize the resources. Peter did not perceive that he had roles to which he could return. After a few years of emotional turmoil, Peter was introduced to a mouth-stick artist who suggested to him that he try to express himself in that medium. Although quite reluctant, he made the attempt and found it to be a meaningful challenge that he was capable of addressing. At that point in time, he began to make use of many of the environmental affordances he previously had ignored. As he developed skill as an artist, he developed self-efficacy that extended beyond his skills with a mouth-stick. He became actively involved with his family once again and returned to school, taking classes in art at a community college. He gradually resumed roles that were typical of other young men, including that of husband and father.

As part of the client's environment, the therapist can provide both affordances and threats. The therapist has innate resources that must be displayed so that the client can identify them. Without the client's apperception of a therapist's resources, they will not become affordances. Additionally, the client must be willing to risk to rely on the therapist in order to take advantage of the resources that are identified as potential affordances. When a client says to a therapist, "I have a lot of confidence in your ability to help me," the client has both identified resources that can become affordances and has determined that the therapist is sufficiently trustworthy that the client will risk depending on those resources. Thus, the affordances of the environment that are tied to the therapist can be used by the client.

CHARACTERISTICS OF THE CLIENT'S ROLE

The primary characteristic of the client's role is that it be meaningful or potentially meaningful. The meaningfulness of the role is based upon the degree to which the accomplishment of the role fits the purpose of the client and the goals that are organized around that purpose. Additionally, the role must be challenging if it is to stimulate the development of competence. Often, roles are not sufficiently stimulating or are overwhelming. In either case, growth does not occur. The role that is not sufficiently stimulating leads to boredom, which is characterized by a generally lower level of energy and gradual erosion of effectancies. Conversely, the role that is overwhelming can lead to decompensation and erosion of self-efficacy with attendant decrease in risk-taking behaviour, exploration, and curiosity. This is seen frequently in rehabilitation as clients attempt new role duties that are challenging. Failure in these attempts is a frequent occurrence. As long as the failure is incorporated as a learning experience and identified as a consequence of remediable factors, decompensation and erosion of self-efficacy will be limited.

The relationship between the meaningfulness of the role and the degree to which it is appropriately challenging is dynamic. That is, to the degree that the role has great meaning for the person, he or she will be willing to entertain a relatively greater level of challenge with the increased risk that is attendant to that challenge because the personal reward is much greater than if the role is less meaningful.

THE NEXUS OF PERSON-ENVIRONMENT ROLE

The interface between effectancies, affordances, and challenges is where competence develops. The therapist can be the steward of this development, but only by being attuned to the client. As noted above, without respect to where the resource originates, each of the resources is uniquely defined by the client. That is, neither affordances, nor challenges, nor effectancies can be fully understood without an understanding of the client. Thus, the therapist must engage the client in ways that will allow the therapist to understand and appreciate the client's perspective.

CHARACTERISTICS OF THE PROFESSIONAL

The professional who is successful in working with the client in occupational therapy must be facilitative of communication. First among the responsibilities is both to listen and to hear the client's communications. Listening is necessary but not sufficient for two reasons. First, listening is necessarily imperfect. None of us completely receives what has been said. Secondly, speaking and other forms of communication are rarely perfect. It is unusual to say exactly what we mean. Clients certainly experience this as well, and must be assisted to communicate with the therapist in a way that allows the therapist to completely understand what the client intends. The process of "active listening" is quite useful in this regard. This requires the listener to provide immediate feedback to the speaker about the listener's understanding of the speaker's communication and to invite clarification. Additionally, the therapist must be facilitative of development of competence in the following ways:

- Improving effectancies through improvement in capacity.
- Improving effectancies through improvement in abilities.
- Improving effectancies through the development of task-relevant skills.
- Identifying available resources that may be affordances.
- Developing resources that can be potential affordances.
- Encouraging the use of resources so that they become affordances.
- Identifying meaningful or potentially meaningful roles.
- Encouraging the attempt to assume a meaningful role.

OUTLINE OF THE DEVELOPMENT PROCESS

The urge toward the competent fulfillment of role demands is a primary human motive. Occupational competence connotes a level of role adequacy in terms of occupational performance. That is, occupational competence is achieved when occupational performance is adequate to role demands. Occupational performance develops to a level of competence in response to challenges that flow from the occupational role demands. Competence is based on the application of effectancies in successful transactions with the environment, using the environmental affordances and responding to the challenges presented by the individual's sociocultural role. Each person configures the match of effectancies and affordances to perform role tasks with optimal self-perceived efficiency. The urge toward competence provides the motivation to facilitate growth, based on self-efficacy beliefs. As successful exploration is sustained, opportunities to develop task competence are identified and attempted so that occupational performance develops to a level of task competence. As task competence aggregates, role competence occurs. The emotionally healthy individual constantly mixes personal and environmental resources to achieve role competence. The therapist's contributions to this process must be guided by the client's goals and willingness to engage in a therapeutic dyad.

ENGAGEMENT AND THE HARNESSING OF MOTIVATION

The client's engagement in the therapeutic process depends on maintaining motivation to develop competence for the identified occupational roles that become the goals of the therapy. Although the techniques that are presented below will be effective to the therapist in most situations, the degree of their effectiveness will be dependent on the ability of the therapist to maintain a client-centred focus and must be undertaken with the full and active acceptance of the client.

INVITATION TO ENGAGE IN THE PROCESS

A characteristic of the client-centred approach that distinguishes it from other approaches is that the initiation of engagement is based on an invitation from the client to the therapist to participate in a relationship. This invitation must be sought by the therapist and must never be presumed to exist. A typical dialogue would be:

Therapist: How can I help you?

Client: I don't know, what do you do?

Therapist: As an occupational therapist, I help people put their lives back together after a serious injury like you have had. Personally, I would enjoy working with you to identify the goals you have related to what you do every day and start working towards them. Is that something you would like some help with?

Client: Yes, but I don't have any idea what my goals are or what I can do.

Therapist: That's OK, the first step is that you want to.

This set of communications from the therapist included both a request for an invitation to participate, and descriptions of both the role of the occupational therapist and a brief description of the therapist's own goals for the relationship. Such a request for an invitation is found in every type of optimally-effective therapeutic relationship, whether it is psychotherapy, occupational therapy, or substance-abuse counseling, to name a few. The client must always invite the therapist to the relationship. This particular interchange resulted in an invitation that allows the process of engagement to unfold. It is also possible that an interchange will not result in an invitation. Consider the following:

Therapist: How can I help you?

Client: I don't want any help.

Therapist: Well, you've been referred to me for therapy. As one of the goals of therapy, it's important to be able to take care of yourself at home, so we'll work on that. Is that something you would like some help with?

Client: Well, I guess I need to be able to take care of myself.

Therapist: Great! Let's get started.

In this interchange, the therapist ignored the declaration of the client and pushed forward to establish a likely therapeutic goal. But, whose goal is this? Perhaps, at some point in time, the client will acquiesce and accept this goal, but an opportunity has been missed to establish a mutually respectful therapeutic relationship that would have been likely to lead to goals in which the client was invested. Let's try again:

Therapist: How can I help you?

Client: I don't want any help.

Therapist: What do you want?

Client: I don't know.

Therapist: That's where most people start.

Client: What do you mean?

Therapist: Most people start without knowing what they want.

Client: What do they do?

Therapist: Different things. Some people talk about what they used to do that they don't think they can do now. Other people focus on getting back to what they were doing before they got hurt. Other people tell me they are so confused they don't know what to think.

The therapist's request for an invitation to engage was rebuffed as a consequence of what was happening in the person who is the client. The therapist's subsequent response, "What do you want?" is client-centred. Later, the description of some of the responses of other people who have been in situations similar to the client's provides affirmation of a wide range of behaviours and helps the client to understand that his or her feelings and possible behaviours are affirmable by the therapist. This affirmation will be lacking for the client in other therapeutic and interpersonal relationships that are not client-centred, thus encouraging the client to move toward a relationship with this therapist. Although not all clients will be willing or able to engage in this process, the client-centred approach to occupational therapy greatly increases the likelihood that meaningful engagement will occur. If it does not, it is important for the therapist to recognize that engagement has not occurred and attempt to identify the cause. If a cause can be identified, the therapist can persevere. It may be that the client is not ready to engage. In that case, it is important for the therapist to monitor the client on a regular basis after seeking and receiving permission to do so. It may also be necessary for the therapist to "hand off" the client to another therapist because the reason for non-engagement may be the therapist's acceptability to the client. This cannot be taken personally by the therapist, nor must the client be identified as difficult or noncooperative. All of us have preferences, the most important of which often involve with whom we like to interact. The client-centred process requires that this be respected by both the client and therapist.

Another value of the client-centred approach to occupational therapy stems from the fact that affirmation provided by the person who is the therapist is more valuable than affirmation provided by the therapist. From the client's perspective, it is certainly more trustworthy in that it can be confirmed by the affective component of the relationship. Further, affirmation of feelings, attitudes, and behaviours will allow the therapist's subsequent affirmation of the client's occupational role competence to be more potent and meaningful to the client.

Optimally, affirmation of the client's occupational role competence occurs in roles that exist beyond the boundaries of the client role, such as parent, spouse, worker, or student. One of the wonderful attributes of occupational therapy is that these nonclient occupational roles are within the purview of the occupational therapist-client dyad. Other professions lack this cachet. The therapist who takes a client-centred approach is much more likely to allow the therapeutic experience to emphasize the importance of occupational role beyond the client role than the therapist who does not.

THE GOALING PROCESS

As discussed in Chapters 5 and 6, an essential part of client-centred practice is having the client identify occupational performance issues that will be goals for therapy. There are a variety of methods to accomplish this. As one method to assist the client to identify, value, and prioritize current goals and to set the stage for the development of additional goals, the goaling process is an excellent introduction. Within a short period of time, this will assist the client to have a firm foundation for planning and a substantially improved understanding of his or her own motives. Goaling helps the client to establish a future orientation, develop a rational basis for planning, and to receive positive feedback from his or her community. This facilitates engagement in therapy by focusing on what is important to the client, creating a "buy in" that is difficult to accomplish otherwise. The goaling process has four steps. Each of the steps must be completed in this order:

1. Structured Interview

The therapist and client meet in a quiet room. In a vocational setting, working with an adult, the therapist asks the client, "What do you want most out of a job?" An inquiry such as, "What do you want most out of retirement?" might be posed to an older person, while an adolescent, might be presented with, "What do you want out of school next year?" The question can be varied to suit the situation, as long as the question requires a future orientation and is role-related. The therapist records the client's responses without comment or judgment, but works with the client to develop individual goal statements that meet the following criteria:

- A goal is a distinct, complete, and clear communication about one issue that makes life more satisfying. Each goal is presented as a complete, but simple, sentence.
- Each goal is listed in its present or future tense.
- Each goal is easily understood and unambiguous.
- Each goal is stated in a positive manner. Negative statements are not recorded. Goals such as "I don't want to make less than $8.00 an hour" or "I don't want to live with my parents" are not acceptable and should be restated in the affirmative. In this example, acceptable goals might be, "I want to earn at least $8.00 an hour" or "I want to live in an apartment on my own."

2. Developing Priorities

Each of the individual goal statements is listed as it is developed by the therapist and the client. After 12 to 15 goals have been identified, the list is presented to the client, and the client is asked to select which of the goals is least important. In fact, all of the goals have importance, but there is an inherent priority that may not be readily apparent to the client. After the client selects the goal that is least important, the therapist continues with the client to select which of the remaining goals is least important. This "negative prioritization" will result in some surprises. At some point during this process, the client may have difficulty in deciding and may state, "All of these are most important." The therapist should persevere and encourage the client to select which of the remaining goals is

---

Table 7-1
Sample Goal List

Goal List for Mary Jones
January 27, 1997

1.   To have health insurance for my children.
2.   To have a safe job.
3.   To have stable employment.
4.   To have good school clothes for my children.
5.   To get my car fixed.
6.   To earn $ 2,200 per month.
7.   To be respected by my children.
8.   To have a strong relationship with God and attend church weekly.
9.   To visit my family in California at least one time each year.
10.   To be respected by my co-workers.
11.   To be a volunteer at my children's school.
12.   To begin dating once again.
13.   To have nice clothes for myself.

---

least important, affirming that all of the goals have importance, but that one of the remaining goals is less important than the others. After this reverse prioritization, a goal list is composed of the goal statements in numerical order from most to least important.

3. Significant Other Review

A copy is made of the prioritized goal list. The original is provided to the client to take home and review with at least one significant other. The client is encouraged to make any changes that may be appropriate in the goals, including adding or deleting goals. The order of the goals may be changed. Wording may be changed. The client is to return with the goal list after a set period of time for this review.

4. Development and Publication of the Goaling Document

After the client returns with the goal list that has been reviewed, a formal list is prepared. An example of a formal goal list appears in Table 7-1.

Twenty copies of the formal goal list are made. The client is provided with the copies and asked to distribute the copies to as many people as he or she can, but no fewer than a certain number negotiated between the therapist and the client. This may be a very challenging experience for the client. It will involve some level of risk and concern about embarrassment. It is also potentially very rewarding. The client is encouraged to provide a goal list to other treating professionals, important family members, friends, and former colleagues or co-workers. One copy should be placed prominently in the client's home, on the refrigerator door or medicine cabinet. The therapist should structure this task so that it is actually completed. The tendency of many clients will be to brush this aspect of the task aside and to not follow through. Experience with several thousand clients has shown that this step is crucial. The client has revealed much of what is important about himself or herself to the therapist. The degree to which the therapist takes the client's goals seriously and respects the client's goals will model the behaviour that the therapist seeks from the client. Similarly, to the degree that the client can appreciate and respect his or her own goals, it will be an important part of the rehabilitation process.

Occupational Self-Exploration

There are several approaches that can be taken to assist the client who is concerned about entering the workforce to explore occupational issues. One of the best strategies for focusing on the vocational aspects of occupational involvement can be accomplished through the use of the Self Directed Search (Holland, 1985). This is a process that the client undertakes using a test booklet and reference guide that can be supplied by the occupational therapist. This is based on the Holland System of Occupational Types (Holland, 1973). John Holland developed a method of classifying the interests of people as they are related to the jobs that people occupy. He developed a system for classification of interests with six different occupational types. These six types can be combined in various ways and are arranged so that they are distinct from each other. This taxonomy has been used in many of the current interest inventories and other methods for classifying the interests that are involved with jobs.

Another approach to assisting the client to identify his or her occupational type and to initiate vocational exploration is through the use of an interest inventory. Depending on how this is presented to the client, it can be a client-centred process, although the experience of participation relies more on the scoring and interpretation of the instrument than is found with the Self Directed Search. Nevertheless, it is a useful approach for therapists who are willing to maintain a client-centred focus in its introduction and administration. The most widely respected of the interest inventories is the Career Assessment Inventory (CAI) (Johansson, 1986). There are several versions of the CAI, each of which is based on the Holland system. These approaches encourage engagement in that they empower the client to easily use widely available information sources about careers and jobs that are organized by this taxonomy.

Functional Capacity, Ability, and Aptitude Testing

The occupational therapist also is able to assist the nurturance of client engagement through exploration of the client's functional capacity, ability, and aptitudes. In fact, this is an important advantage that the occupational therapist has over most other types of health care professionals. In the vocational area, this is usually accomplished through formal testing, such as a Functional Capacity Evaluation or Work Capacity Evaluation. The degree to which the therapist can facilitate the client's development in this area will depend on the therapist's academic preparation and professional training. Many of these instruments are controlled by their publishers, based on criteria that are intended to ensure that the test administrator is competent. References for the therapist can be found in Asher (1996) and Matheson (1996). Functional evaluation is a type of intervention that can encourage engagement if it is used to educate the client in terms of what he or she can do, rather than focus on loss or limitation of ability.

Coupled with testing to uncover and affirm abilities, vocational exploration can be facilitated by the occupational therapist in several ways. Use of references such as the *Occupational Outlook Handbook* (U.S. Department of Labor, 1996) along with results of the goaling process, occupational exploration, and functional, ability, and aptitude testing can greatly facilitate the client's identification of vocational options. These vocational options can be considered in terms of the goals and resources of the client and can become the basis of a formal rehabilitation plan. A plan that is derived in this way is so strongly client-centred that it is likely to maintain the interest, active involvement, and motivation of the client at the same time that it recruits the assistance of family members, care providers, and the agencies that underwrite payment for rehabilitation.

The person-centred approach to occupational therapy can be facilitated by therapeutic techniques and assessment processes that promote engagement and self-exploration. The primary characteristics of successful engagement of this type are that it flows from the needs of the client, expressed within a client-centred therapeutic dyad in which mutual trust and respect have been developed. Such relationships are difficult to achieve in many professional contexts of practice. Nevertheless, these relationships are worthy and capable vehicles for potent therapeutic effect that captures the client as a person. As a consequence, client-centred engagement will generalize across all interventions to potentiate and extend the effects of rehabilitation.

REFERENCES

Asher, I. (1996). *Occupational therapy assessment tools: An annotated index.* Bethesda, MD: American Occupational Therapy Association.

Bandura, A. (1989). Human agency in social cognitive theory.*American Psychologist 44,* 1175-1184.

Bandura, A. (1990). Conclusion: Reflections on Nonability Determinant of CompetenceIn R. Sternberg & J. Kolligian (Eds.). *Competence considered.* New Haven, CT: Yale University Press.

Baum, C. (1991). Identification and use of environmental resources. In C. Christiansen & C. Baum (Eds.). *Occupational therapy: Overcoming human performance deficits.* Thorofare, NJ: SLACK Incorporated.

Beck, A. (1976). *Cognitive therapy and emotional disorders.* New York: New American Library.

Ellis, A. (1979). *Reason and emotion in psychotherapy.* New York: Stuart.

Holland, J. (1973). *Making vocational choices: a theory of careers.* Englewood Cliffs, NJ: Prentice-Hall.

Holland, J. (1985). *The self-directed search.* Odessa, FL: Psychological Assessment Resources.

Johansson, C. (1986). *Career assessment inventory.* Minneapolis, MN: National Computer Systems.

Kirschenbaum, H., Henderson, V. (Eds.) (1989). *The Carl Rogers Reader.* New York: Houghton Mifflin.

Maslow, A. (1968). *Toward a psychology of being.* Princeton, NJ: Van Nostrand.

Maslow, A. (1971). *The farther reaches of human nature.* New York: Viking.

Matheson, L. (1996). Functional capacity evaluation. In G. Andersson, S. Demeter, & G. Smith (Eds.). *Disability evaluation.* St. Louis: Mosby Yearbook.

Matheson, L., & Bohr, P. (1997). In C. Christiansen & M. Baum (Eds.). *Occupational therapy: Enabling performance and well-being.* Thorofare, NJ: SLACK Incorporated.

Rogers, C. (1961). *On becoming a person.* Boston: Houghton Mifflin.

Rogers, C. (1980). *A way of being*. Boston: Houghton Mifflin.

Seligman, M. (1975). *Helplessness: On depression, development and death*. New York: W. H. Freeman.

Seligman, M. (1991). *Learned optimism*. New York: A. A. Knopf.

U. S. Department of Labor (1996). *Occupational outlook handbook*. Washington, DC: United States Government Printing Office.

White, R. (1959). Motivation reconsidered: the concept of competence. *Psychoanalytic Review, 66*, 197.

White, R. (1971). The urge towrds competence. *American Journal of Occupational Therapy, 25*(6), 271-274.

White, R. (1974). Strategies of adaptation: An attempt at systematic description. In G. Coelho, D. Hamburg, & J. Adams (Eds.). *Coping and adaptation*. New York: Basic Books.

CLIENT-CENTRED OCCUPATIONAL THERAPY: COLLABORATIVE PLANNING, ACCOUNTABLE INTERVENTION

KAREN WHALLEY HAMMELL, MSc, OT(C)

This chapter will focus on methods of ensuring that what happens during occupational therapy intervention reflects the principles of client-centred practice. "Intervention" in occupational therapy is the process of working to effect change in an aspect of occupational performance using meaningful occupations (Canadian Association of Occupational Therapists, 1997). This chapter explores intervention in relation to process and with regard to the values underpinning this process. A "process" is "a state of being in progress, a narrative, a series of actions and events, and a sequence of changes undergone" (*Chambers Twentieth Century Dictionary*, 1972). This dynamic course is informed by the values that necessitate a client-centred approach to practice: regard for client values, support for success and risk, facilitation of client-identified needs, and open communication with reciprocal exchange of information.

The philosophical approach to intervention that client-centred practice symbolizes is concerned with ensuring the meaningfulness of intervention. In this chapter, the process of occupational therapy intervention will be related to the context and meaning of disability through consideration of biography, biographical disruption, and narrative. Goal planning, motivation, ethics, autonomy, and contemporary adult learning theory underlie the rehabilitation process. Intervention and outcome measurement are inextricably linked and will be considered in relation to how principles of client-centredness might inform outcome measurement and programme evaluation. Fundamentally, client-centred occupational therapy intervention is dependent upon an exchange of information: a theme that recurs throughout this chapter.

UNDERSTANDING THE CONTEXT FOR OCCUPATIONAL THERAPY INTERVENTION

Rehabilitation programmes have traditionally sought to teach skills and to develop strategies for intervention that are often unrelated to the life-world of the individual, but which adhere to a predetermined schedule (Hammell, 1995a). Thus, instead of addressing those abilities "necessary to maintain one's self in day-to-day routines and demands," (Keith, 1995, p. 77) clients have been taught skills that are quickly discarded as irrelevant in a real-world context (Rogers & Figone, 1980; Weingarden & Martin, 1989; Yerxa &

Locker, 1990). Clients may share a diagnosis with other clients, but interventions must be applicable to the unique environment, life stage, and goals of the individual and must consider the meaning that the disability holds for him or her and the place of that disability within his or her biography.

Sociologists have suggested that a disease or disability may be viewed as an "interrupted life trajectory" (Strauss & Glasser, 1975). This provides a useful metaphor in that it invokes the sense of a life in progress, with continuity, a past, and a future. Illness or disability has also been characterised as a disruptive biographical experience, wherein the routine activity and structure of everyday life is disordered (Bury, 1982). This biographical disruption demands conscious attention to life plans, habits, goals, values, and meanings. In particular, there is a loss of the taken-for-granted nature of the life-world of the individual. Conceptualised by philosophers Husserl and Schütz, the life-world refers to the "realm of beliefs, assumptions, values, and cultural practices that constitute meaning in everyday life" (Kögler, 1995, p. 488-489).

Ethnographic accounts suggest the tremendous effort that older people expend in an attempt to maintain and preserve their past identities and continue these into the future. Aware of their devalued status in the eyes of society, they seek to demonstrate continuity with their past lives by recalling and asserting former identities based, perhaps, in occupation, family, or parenting (Cohen, 1994). This concern with biographical continuity is echoed by Giddens (1991) who proposes that the self seeks to connect the individual's past and future lives through its authorship of a narrative project. This process of biographical continuity and reconstruction takes place within a social context and has important implications for occupational therapy intervention.

OCCUPATION, BIOGRAPHY, AND BIOGRAPHICAL DISRUPTION: CONTEXT AND MEANING

Corbin and Strauss (1987) propose three major dimensions of biography: the body, conceptions of self and identity, and biographical time (temporal adaptation): issues central to occupational therapy. A basic assumption of occupational therapy is that engagement in occupations, or one's daily configuration of activities, is related to life satisfaction (Yerxa & Baum, 1986). Occupations are defined as "use of time, energy, interest and attention," (Wilcock, 1993, p. 1) are performed within a social and cultural context, and are imbued with personal meaning (Law, 1991). Indeed, it is proposed that identity is expressed through "the enactment of occupations and the narrative interpretation associated with those occupations" (Jackson, 1995, p. 676).

Extending the metaphor of biographical disruption, as illness, injury, or disability interrupts or destroys life plans, projects, and habitual patterns of activity, people speak of the need for "authorship" of their activities and a reassertion of control over their lives. It is suggested that people gain a sense of control by "choosing, shaping and orchestrating" their daily occupations (Clark & Jackson, 1989, p. 74). Bury (1991) proposes that meaning and context cannot easily be separated when considering biography. Experiences are influenced by the context of the individual's life and the unique social, cultural, physical, economic, political, and legal environment (Health Services Directorate and the Canadian Association of Occupational Therapists, 1993; McColl, Law, & Stewart, 1993) that serves to shape the experience and meaning of illness or disability.

Viewing an illness or disability as a disruptive biographical event encourages occupational therapists to consider the meaning of the disruption in the life history of the individual and his or her family. Thus, interventions will not be directed solely toward a biological state but to the human world of motives, values, beliefs, and the meaning that the disability holds for the individual. The person who has sustained a stroke, severe head injury, or spinal cord injury (for example) has permanently disrupted an entire life (Mattingly, 1991a). Biographical reconstruction aims to bring continuity and meaning to life, such that illness or disability is integrated into the fabric of life, becoming part of the texture of a biography rather than its central theme (Corbin & Strauss, 1987). Rather than focusing predominantly on the interrelated issues of disruption and loss, it is suggested that a more useful strategy is for the occupational therapist to help the client identify and address dimensions of continuity.

In a recent study of people with high-level spinal cord injuries, the theme of continuity recurred repeatedly. People spoke of the support of family members who recognised that they were the same people as before their injuries and who saw no restrictions to what could be accomplished, encouraging them to live a normal lifestyle, to take risks, and to pursue former interests within the parameters of their limitations. As an occupational therapist, it was embarrassing to note the contrast that was made between the attitude of families, who encouraged exploration of opportunities and facilitated risk-taking, and that of their health care professionals, who were depicted as universally pessimistic (Hammell, 1997).

This demonstrates the crucial role of the family in rehabilitation. It is not difficult to extrapolate Bury's theory to consider the biographical disruption experienced by others close to the person with the disability. Rehabilitation practitioners have frequently been criticised for focusing all their attention on the needs of one, clearly identified client, while ignoring or overlooking the interrelated needs of, for example, partners, parents, or children. Client-centred practice does not demand that attention and intervention be focused on only one client. Those closely impacted by the disability, exacerbation, or other life-event may also be clients whose inter-related needs must be considered as part of the intervention process.

BIOGRAPHY AND NARRATIVE

There is a growing body of interdisciplinary literature suggesting that narratives provide a powerful way of understanding dimensions of human motives and actions (Helfrich, Kielhofner, & Mattingly, 1994). Narrative is a form in which experience is represented and recounted, and activities are described along with the significance that lends them their meaning for those involved (Good, 1994). "Challenged personal narratives" (Helfrich & Kielhofner, 1994, p. 321) (disrupted biographies) require clients to reconstruct, reaffirm, redirect, or otherwise continue their life-stories into the future. Rich in contextualisation, narratives provide a framework for understanding how the experience of disability is shaped within social and cultural frameworks, the meanings that underlie observed behaviour, and the purpose of therapy and goals within that life (Robinson, 1990; Monks & Frankenberg, 1995). "Narratives make sense of reality by linking the outward world of actions and events to the inner world of human intention and motivation" (Mattingly, 1991b, p. 999). Attention to narrative shifts the focus of intervention from the physical or emotional "problem" to the meaning and impact of that problem within a life.

Kielhofner and Mallinson (1995) provide some useful guidelines for facilitating narratives within the context of an interview. Informal, semi-structured interviewing techniques are routinely used by occupational therapists, and attention to certain modes of questioning can elicit narrative responses that provide a depth of insight into the values and meanings that inform the client's interpretation of events. Questions concerning changes in the direction of life, for example, may provoke narrative data concerning the significance of life events and the meaning of these for the client, thereby providing insight into values and motivators. Successful intervention will be dependent upon aligning the therapist's perspective with that of the client and this can clearly be facilitated by use of narrative questioning, even within the context of acute-care or short-term settings. Collaborative planning for intervention should consider the social roles and expectations of each individual, their relationships, cultural and environmental context, and how these factors will inform the activities that are continued or given up in the presence of a disability.

Helfrich and Kielhofner (1994, p. 321) demonstrate how attention to a client's narrative provides insight into the meaning of occupational therapy intervention, describing how a journalist struggling with manic depressive illness experienced occupational therapy activities as "humiliating detours," more appropriate to his life as a patient than to his return to a life in the community. Mattingly (1994) describes each encounter between client and therapist as an episode in a therapeutic narrative, a short story within the larger life story of the client.

Williams (1987, p. 98) suggests that "the disruption of habitual activity by disability undermines the web of meaning that gives coherence to everyday life." It is this "web of meaning" that lies undetected in traditional forms of assessment upon which interventions have been based. Occupational therapists will treat what they assess. If assessments are based upon self-care skills, these will be the sole focus for intervention, irrespective of the value of these activities to the individual. Client-centred assessment attained through use of a tool that encourages or facilitates narrative, such as the Canadian Occupational Performance Measure (COPM) (Law, Baptiste, Carswell, Polatajko, & Pollock, 1994), will ascertain client-identified problems, focus upon the client's sociocultural, organisational, and physical environment, and consider the client's satisfaction with present performance (Law, Baptiste, Carswell, Polatajko, & Pollock, 1994). If assessments are focused in this way upon the individual's unique biography, his or her goals, roles, and values, it is more likely that the therapy programme will be directed toward the individual's life rather than his or her emotional or physical status (Hammell, 1994a, 1994b).

SPIRITUALITY: BIOGRAPHY AND MEANING

Occupational therapists have had a traditional and predominant preoccupation with self-care activities to the comparative neglect of occupations concerned with leisure or productivity (Hammell, 1995a). Perhaps this reflects a belief that life satisfaction or the experience of quality of life is closely related to the ability to perform self-care tasks. This would presuppose that a high degree of physical independence (or lesser degree of disability) would be positively correlated with high life satisfaction. However, studies of people with physical disabilities have found that there is no relationship between the severity of disability (or degree of physical independence) and life satisfaction (Abela & Dijkers, 1994; Cushman & Hassett, 1992; Fuhrer, 1996; Fuhrer, Rintala, Hart, Clearman, & Young, 1992; Kirchman, 1986; Krause & Dawis, 1992; Lindberg, 1995; Nosek, Fuhrer, & Potter, 1995; Siösteen, Lundqvist, Blomstrand, Sullivan, & Sullivan, 1990; Crisp, 1992; Whiteneck, Charlifue, & Frankel, 1992). Indeed, suicide rates are higher among people with incomplete spinal cord lesions or those with paraplegia than among those with higher lesions and more profound physical impairments (DeVivo, Black, Richards, & Stover, 1991). Further, there is more research evidence supporting the influence of occupation on health in areas of work and leisure than in the area of self-care (Law, Steinwender, & LeClair, In press). It could, therefore, be argued that it is not the physical dimension of a disability that dictates outcome, nor is life satisfaction predicted by the ability to perform self-care skills independently. Rather, it is the psychosocial issues of living with a disability in a unique environment, within an individual biography, imbued with personal meaning. Accordingly, Trieschmann (1988) suggests that the rehabilitation team should not only focus on the acquisition of skills to enable clients to get out of bed in the morning, but should also assist them in finding their own reasons for so doing.

Occupational therapists have identified spirituality as one of the fundamental elements underpinning occupational therapy practice. Spirituality has been defined by occupational therapists as "the experience of meaning in everyday life" (Urbanowski & Vargo, 1994, p. 89). Consideration of spirituality "acknowledges that humans reflect on the nature and meaning of their lives" (Health Services Directorate and the Canadian Association of Occupational Therapists, 1993, p. 7). Campbell (Osbon, 1991, p. 16) has observed that the meaning of life is whatever one brings to it, "whatever you ascribe it to be." Thus, humans define the meaning they experience *in* their lives. Sartre, the existentialist philosopher, argued that the biological, psychological, social, and economic circumstances of an individual are contingent facts of life but that, as a conscious being, the individual chooses what meaning is given to these facts (Lavine, 1984). Occupational therapists recognize that spirituality arises both from within an individual and from environmental forces that influence individuals in defining their own meanings (Canadian Association of Occupational Therapists, 1994).

Kirsh (1996) has illustrated how a narrative approach to occupational therapy intervention enables an understanding of how clients experience meaning and purpose in their lives, emphasizing the need to discover personal meaning in life. It is this dimension of meaning that occupational therapy intervention must seek to address.

COLLABORATIVE PLANNING FOR OCCUPATIONAL THERAPY INTERVENTION

Collaborative goal setting (as described in Chapter 5) by client and occupational therapist ensures that the programme of intervention is directed toward mastering skills that the client values and is likely to use. It further enables analysis of whether intervention should appropriately be targeted at changes in the client (such as learning time management skills) or the environment (such as advocating for nondiscriminatory access to public transportation) (Hammell, 1995a; Jongbloed & Crichton, 1990; Hammell, 1994c). The philosophy underlying client-centred intervention is compatible with that of the Independent Living Movement, a cross-disability social movement of people who aim to attain social justice and achieve full control over their own lives. The Independent Living Movement has some basic underlying principles, including consumer choice of service delivery, the "right to risk" as an inherent component of true independence and self-determination, and the right of all people to direct their own lives and choose their own lifestyles (Oxelgren, Harker, Hammell, & Boyes, 1992).

Sadly, the literature contains many examples of discordance between clients' and therapists' goals. An early study examined the occupational therapy goals of people with paraplegia and quadriplegia and those of their occupational therapists. The therapists and their clients identified quite different goals, the discrepancy between the people with quadriplegia and their therapists being especially marked (Taylor, 1974). A recent study that examined the psychosocial situation of people with head injury or spinal cord injury living in the community identified the divergence that had commonly been experienced between the intervention goals of therapists and their clients. One wife commented, "They thought at the Spinal Centre that the important thing was to be able to transfer. He still can't—but it doesn't matter. He's happy and I'm happy. There are more important things" (Hammell, 1991).

Her husband agreed that he had neither desire nor need to transfer by himself. Transferring was a skill he did not plan to learn but that his therapists believed he should learn. This represents a considerable opportunity cost and further raises the issue of accountability. Clearly, the therapists were neither accountable to the client (whose express wishes they attempted to over-rule), nor to the funding agency, which was required to fund professional time spent in futile endeavours. It would clearly have been more useful to learn something of the life-world of this client (his very comfortable financial situation and exceptional family support, which effectively eliminated his need to perform transfers alone) in addition to his own interpretation of his situation (he informed the researcher that his overwhelming fear of falling from his chair prohibited any inclination to transfer on his own). A reframing of this encounter could, without much difficulty, have informed a therapy programme directed toward his life-world, values, and goals.

THERAPEUTIC RELATIONSHIPS: PROCESS AND PARTNERSHIPS

An effort to achieve clinical practice that is grounded in the daily realities of our clients' lives and that addresses client-identified problems demands that the occupational therapist relinquish the posture of an expert. This neither requires nor allows the therapist to surrender responsibility, but, rather, it requires more emphasis on "process," that is, upon interaction, negotiation, communication, and exchange of information. Peloquin (1990) describes a therapeutic interaction in which the therapist fosters a relationship founded on reciprocity and characterised by trust, commitment, and respect. This relationship encourages the client to use the therapist as a resource while enabling the therapist to understand the concerns of the client. This maximizes the skills and resources of the occupational therapist, who must draw upon experiential and academic knowledge in enabling the client to envision possibilities and establish valued goals.

Occupational therapy may usefully be viewed as an event interpenetrating a person's biography. In the infamous autobiographical chapter entitled "I didn't come here to bake cookies," Rick Hansen describes the occupational therapy programme designed for him as a 15 year old. Baking cookies was not an activity compatible with his goals or relevant to the meaning of paralysis within his teenage life, and he did not participate (Hansen & Taylor, 1988). Similarly, the anthropologist Robert Murphy (1987) described the impact of disease and paralysis upon his own life and reported that he did well in occupational therapy, although he considered some of the activities to be "ridiculous." It must surely be disrespectful to expect participation in activities that lack meaning, relevance, or reward.

Concerns have been expressed that client-centred intervention will demand more time from therapists than would a therapist-centred model of practice. The previous examples serve to illustrate a contrary notion: that effective use of therapists' time may, in reality, be less costly, requiring less input and enhancing accountability.

People with spinal cord injuries have expressed frustration at the inability to "contribute" following injury and have linked this ability to the sense of having value and being valued (Hammell, 1997). A former client with paraplegia elected to construct a large wooden newspaper stand for his roommate in the rehabilitation centre, a young man with high quadriplegia. This task provided the opportunity to increase balance and strengthen the upper body while enabling participation in an activity that was both meaningful and rewarding and that generated a sense of value.

A British study examined the experiences of people discharged from a National Spinal Injuries Centre (Oliver, Zarb, Silver, Moore, & Salisbury, 1988). Several people described a rehabilitation process so regimental that the programme might have been "engraved in tablets of stone" (p. 24); each individual was expected to "slot in" (p. 24). One person commented that rehabilitation was "like a conveyor belt" (p. 79), and another said "it was standard procedure to do certain things" (p. 79). Overall, it was felt that "responsiveness to individual preferences would go some way to improving the adequacy of the occupational therapy service" (p. 80). The most positive response in the study was intriguing. One former client described how his therapist had the confidence to relinquish power and control and to view their joint participation as a partnership. Although claiming to have been "a difficult patient" (p. 80) (because he had a clear idea of what he wanted to accomplish!), he explained that they had worked together to solve his problems (Oliver, Zarb, Silver, Moore, & Salisbury, 1988).

It may be argued that an occupational therapy service, by definition, has a different underlying philosophy than that espoused by some other services. While occupational therapy directs interventions toward "activities specifically related to occupational performance in the areas of self-care, productivity and leisure" (Health Services Directorate and the Canadian Association of Occupational Therapists, 1993), other services target performance components, which, by their nature, tend to be decontextualized from the client's life-world. Further, the success of occupational therapy intervention is dependent upon an understanding of the complex relationship between the individual's impairment, the social context within which the impairment is experienced, and the meanings available to the individual to make sense of this experience.

Providing more flexibility in enabling clients access to occupational therapy services on a long-term basis has the potential to provide a more responsive intervention and would relieve therapists of the fear that clients had not learned every essential skill before returning to the community. This could be facilitated by enhanced self-referral and by follow-up appointments held in the context of the client's environment rather than that of the therapists. Therapists' preference for regular work schedules effectively prohibits outpatient attendance by clients who themselves have employment or educational commitments. A more flexible service, with therapists available on weekends and during evenings would help to meet the client's agenda: a client-centred approach to institutional organization (Hammell, 1995a).

COOPERATION AND COMPLIANCE, OR COLLABORATION AND AUTONOMY?

Rehabilitation staff have traditionally favoured client compliance with policies, routines, and interventions. However, compliance may not be in the best interest of the client. Compliance is not an attribute that best serves the individual in achieving meaningful goals, and cooperation does not predict independent living success after discharge (Hammell, 1995a). Compliance with externally imposed routines does not enable the person to assume responsibility for his or her health, facilitate problem-solving, or encourage self-directive behaviour (Tucker, 1984; Trieschmann, 1986). Indeed, if the client is neither permitted to define his or her own problems nor to engage in a problem-solving process, the overwhelming sense of powerlessness and loss of self-determination may, in fact, appear as noncompliance (Pollock, 1993).

For some people, personal-care skills will be a primary goal during rehabilitation, and every effort will be made to match the client's abilities and potential with equipment and techniques to achieve this goal. Other clients may have different living environments in physical, social, cultural, and economic terms, preferring to share tasks with others and use time and energy for goals related to other occupations (Hammell, 1995a). Without a clear understanding of the client's biography, cultural background, socioeconomic situation, and value system to inform goal planning, the therapist is unlikely to be able to foresee exactly what precise skills the client will need.

I have proposed that occupational therapy intervention must be meaningful to the individual and that intervention planning must be a collaborative process. Brief examples from published accounts have lent weight to this argument. However, therapists have queried this approach in instances where a client refuses to participate in learning self-care skills that the therapist believes to be important. Traditionally, outcome assessment has measured what clients can do rather than what they actually do, thus therapists' intervention programmes may have appeared highly successful, if not highly relevant. However, research studies that have examined those self-care skills actually undertaken following discharge have reported findings that represent a reordering of time and energy based on personal priorities. Many individuals discontinue their efforts to maintain physical independence in self-care, choosing to engage in more satisfying pursuits (Rogers & Figone, 1980; Weingarden & Martin, 1989; Yerxa & Baum, 1986; Yerxa & Locker, 1990).

INTERVENTION INFORMED BY BIOGRAPHY

The therapists' skills and knowledge are maximised in sharing information and experience concerning the possibilities and opportunities that may be available and achievable for each client. Rohe and Athelstan (1982, 1985) studied the vocational interests of people who had recently sustained spinal cord injuries, following up their study after some years had elapsed. At an average of eight years after injury, people with spinal cord injuries had increased their level of interest in the arts and in areas of social involvement. It was also found that the interests that were present before injury did not diminish. The researchers propose, therefore, that rehabilitation professionals should assess former interests, assume that these interests are unlikely to change greatly, "and help devise strategies for acting on interests that are present but no longer physically possible" (Rohe & Athelstan, 1985, p. 141). This ensures that intervention is informed by the client's biography.

The popular press provide a high-profile illustration. Following actor Christopher Reeve's high spinal cord injury, he has refocused his energies and interest in the entertainment industry, providing the voice for a cartoon character and directing a drama for television (Entertainment Weekly, 1996). A young man who sustained a similar injury playing ice hockey refocused his time and talent by reviewing videotapes of his team's games and assisting his former coach in devising future game plans. This enabled him to maximise the time he had to spend in bed and encouraged him to feel that he could still make a valuable contribution to his team and to the game he loved. The occupational therapist was involved in the selection of a suitable environmental control unit that would enable independent operation of the functions of a videocassette player and television.

Ozer (1988) outlines a process to help engage client participation in planning intervention. He suggests that the therapist commence by asking in general terms what the client hopes to gain from the particular intervention, thereby enabling the client to identify goals and concerns. Should this strategy fail, the therapist can take a multiple choice line of questioning from which the client selects an answer. If this approach is unsuccessful, the therapist can suggest an answer, and ask the client to agree or disagree. Ozer proposes that the planning process should always allow maximum choice to elicit client participation and only if this fails should the multiple or forced options be tried. At no time is "no choice" advocated, wherein the client complies with a plan predetermined by someone else.

Ozer's approach has been documented in the process of choosing a powered wheelchair (Curtin & Clarke, 1997) and in determining learning needs in the computer resource room (Curtin & Powell, 1997). In the latter example, the therapist provided an initial training period to introduce the technology, and clients were encouraged thereafter to play an active role in planning and directing what they wanted to do, based upon interests, needs, and goals. The therapist encouraged the clients to compare and evaluate the various access options, to identify their own problems, locate information, decide on a course of action and evaluate consequences. The therapists, thereby, facilitated a process of problem-based learning in which the client was encouraged to identify a "question" and assume responsibility for finding the answer (Hammell, 1995a, 1995b).

Such a collaborative approach may appear solely relevant to adults with physical disabilities. However, striking similarities have been identified between the needs and demands of people with physical, psychiatric, and developmental disabilities, most particularly the wish for control and self-determination and the need to engage in meaningful activities and roles (Pentland, Krupa, Lynch, & Clark, 1992). People with psychiatric disabilities, for example, will function at a lower level in a setting with low stimulation and few challenges than when tasks are perceived as real and personally meaningful. Studies have suggested, however, that clients and professionals tend to identify very different needs. "In a system where the professional alone is ascribed the credibility, the result may be that individuals are separated from control over their lives" (Pentland, Krupa, Lynch, & Clark, 1992, p. 129). Clearly, this is the reverse of what occupational therapy ostensibly aims to achieve.

Few occupational therapists have an intimate understanding of what it means to live with a disability in the community. Certainly, this has been the complaint of some former clients (Hammell, 1991). Models of service delivery should enable responsive professional support in the community as new problems are encountered or the need for new skills or equipment is identified. This would provide a more reflexive service to clients and an opportunity for therapists to learn more of what disability means within the context of their clients' lives (Hammell, 1995a, 1995b). Service provision centred within the client's environment would also facilitate involvement of family members and friends. If rehabilitation is construed as the process of learning to live with a disability in the context of one's own environment (Trieschmann, 1988), it could reasonably be proposed that this is the most appropriate context within which to frame occupational therapy intervention. Attention to meaning demands consideration of the unique environment within which meaning is shaped and activities are experienced as purposeful.

MOTIVATION

Active collaboration of client and therapist requires commitment, respect, engagement, and motivation. Recent writers have articulated a perspective on motivation that is particularly pertinent to client-centred philosophy. Traditionally viewed as an inner drive, "lack of motivation" has been a derogatory descriptor for someone who does not cooperate with treatment regimens. The client labeled "unmotivated" has been viewed as a failure, as unambitious and a time-waster (Hammell, 1995a). One published report cites the case of a woman who was referred for psychiatric consultation because she was "failing to meet either the short- or long-term goals established for her by our hospital's Rehabilitation Unit" (Steinglass, Temple, Lisman, & Reiss, 1982, p. 261). It is worth considering whose values, needs, and priorities had underpinned these goals and whether a re-evaluation of the goals would have been a more appropriate and respectful course of action. Problems may not always originate with the client (Hammell, 1995a).

Researchers have begun to examine the environment as a critical element in the assessment of motivation. According to contemporary philosophy, people who are unmotivated to participate actively in their rehabilitation programmes are those for whom rehabilitation is offering no rewards for which they choose to work. Further, if a client has learned that goals and interventions are determined by other, more powerful people, he or she is less likely to work hard toward attaining these goals. Client goal choice has been described as a "potent motivational construct" (Cook, 1981, p. 11). It is conversely suggested that motivation may be blunted by differences in client-therapist perspectives toward goals, indeed, "treatment environments can override client goals and result in ineffective rehabilitation" (Cook, 1981, p. 11).

Motivation is frequently equated with cooperation, with the implicit assumption that if someone is cooperating with the therapists' objectives, he or she must be well-motivated. By default, an uncooperative person will be labeled unmotivated. In reality, however, the client may be highly motivated to work toward valued goals, but may reject the definition that others have made of his or her problems and their perceptions of what appropriate goals should be (Hammell, 1995a).

It is suggested that "motivational levels will be low if the 'change cost'—the amount of physical or psychological effort required to effect change—is disproportionate to the client's value of the potential outcome" (Hammell, 1994a, p. 47).

This implies that an occupational therapy goal or activity that has little value to the client and to his or her evaluation of its importance to life will be likely to result in low motivation and a poor outcome (Jordan, Wellborn, Kovnik, & Saltzstein, 1991). Abberley (1995, p. 227) observes that occupational therapists are typically involved in a process of adjusting the client's view of reality to match that of the therapist: "In OT theory this process is seen as educational." Examples in the literature suggest the futility of interventions based on therapists' priorities. In establishing goals that are meaningful to the client and worth his or her considerable change cost, it is clearly essential that occupational therapists understand the client's own concerns, values, and goals and the impact and meaning of the disability within his or her life (Hammell, 1995a). It may thus be proposed that realignment of power in the assessment and intervention planning processes toward a truly collaborative model may serve to enhance levels of motivation—for both members of the partnership.

"Motivation... is linked to spirituality and recognises the necessity of eliciting and sustaining human volition as a basis for action" (Health Services Directorate and the Canadian Association of Occupational Therapists, 1993, p. 7).

Occupational therapists attempt to utilize therapeutic activities that provide a balance between challenge and skills. It has been observed that the quality of the experience of engagement in an activity will be the most positive when the client perceives that the challenge posed by the environment is matched by his or her capacity to act (skill) (Csikszentmihalyi, 1993; Csikszentmihalyi & LeFevre, 1989).

This process has been described by a man with a C1 quadriplegia as follows:

"It wasn't like I was going to set the world on fire—you just find some sort of challenge and it really keeps you occupied ... I just took small steps—but I took a lot of small steps ... Keep it small and then keep building on each one of those successes—and that's how my dreams became bigger and bigger." (Hammell, 1997)

LEARNED/TAUGHT HELPLESSNESS

The theory of learned helplessness states that, unless people feel able to exert some control over their lives and events, they will cease making the effort to try to do so (Seligman, 1975). If the treatment environment demands cooperative, compliant, and passive behaviour from a client, this will contribute to a sense of powerlessness in which the client is taught to depend upon professional experts for goal identification, intervention planning, and decision-making related to the disability. This could more appropriately be termed taught helplessness, thus locating its source with the teachers rather than the learners (Hammell, 1995a).

Occupational therapists have viewed independence as a worthy rehabilitation goal. Unfortunately, this has usually been narrowly defined as physical independence in self-care skills. I offer the following definitions of independence: not subordinate, completely self-governing, thinking or acting for oneself (*Chambers Twentieth Century Dictionary*, 1972). An independent individual is one who can identify problems, establish plans and work toward them, and, if necessary, direct others in his or her care (Hammell, 1995a). Independence may thus be viewed as a state of mind rather than a physical ability, an attribute fostered by active engagement in planning goals, ordering priorities, and monitoring progress. Taught helplessness is iatrogenic and the antithesis of successful rehabilitation. Thus, lack of meaningful activity and social isolation have been identified as factors contributing to learned helplessness in long-term care environments. The "iatrogenic diseases of institutional life" (Lorimer, 1984, p. 62) may be alleviated by such measures as encouraging individual choice in furnishings and meal times, and establishing resident committees and empowering them with decision-making responsibilities (Lorimer, 1984).

It is suggested that seniors may be especially susceptible to developing learned helplessness behaviours, characterised by depression, powerlessness, and disengagement (Hooker, 1986). Decreased tolerance to fatigue may be compounded by increased difficulty learning new skills, habits, and behaviours (Hammell, 1995a). However, the philosophy of client-centred practice is no less important for the older client. McKinnon (1992) reports that Canadian seniors use 7.5 hours per day for leisure activities, hence occupational therapy intervention may be predominantly devoted to exploration of leisure interests and opportunities for socialisation. Early collaboration in identifying meaningful goals and activities will help to reduce the tendency toward helplessness and dependence upon staff (Hammell, 1995a).

CLIENT-CENTRED PRACTICE AND THE TEACHING-LEARNING PROCESS

Adult education requires the learner to be an active participant in an interactive process, not the passive recipient of a list of information or skills. Education is about imparting the confidence to pose a question and about imparting the responsibility to find the answer; hence, learning will only be successful if it is concerned with clients' own perceptions of their needs and goals (Hammell, 1995b). Therapists have complained, "We tried to teach them, but they didn't learn" (McVeigh, 1989, p. 263). In reality, these clients may have rebelled against a learning experience perceived as being devoid of value or relevance (Jordan, Wellborn, Kovnik, & Saltzstein, 1991).

The process of education must be as much about teaching the therapist what disability means to the individual as it is about helping the client learn how to attain a rewarding and fulfilling lifestyle (Hammell, 1995b). It has been proposed that professional competence has two components. One dimension is a sound grasp of the techniques or formal knowledge of the profession; the other aspect is "the ability to enter the patient's life-world so that the techniques are tailored to meet the patient's needs" (Crepeau, 1991, p. 1024). Acknowledging that each client has a different life-world and, thus, a unique perspective on the experience of disability, Crepeau (1991) describes one session of occupational therapy intervention: an interaction as concerned with teaching the therapist about the experience of quadriplegia as it was about teaching the client how to function with quadriplegia. The therapist did not seek to impose her definition of the problem on the client, but rather created opportunities for the client to teach her about his own interpretations, meanings, and experience. Crepeau demonstrates how the therapist engaged her client in an activity that enabled practice using a tenodesis grip and that encouraged the development of balance in sitting, while maintaining a dialogue informed by her own prior knowledge. By sharing her previous experience and insights while simultaneously encouraging the client to express his interpretations and experiences, both client and therapist were able to test and revise their knowledge schemata (Crepeau, 1991).

Traditionally, knowledge viewed as being objective, neutral, or scientific was accorded privilege over expertise derived from lived experience. Client-centred practice attempts to utilise both forms of knowledge: the experiential knowledge of the client and the academic and practical knowledge of the therapist. Schön (1983) urges health care professionals to encourage a reflective dialogue with a client in order to place knowledge into the framework and context of the individual's life and experiences.

It has been suggested that people learn best when they are helped to define their own problems, decide on a course of action and, most importantly, evaluate the consequences of their decisions (Coles, 1989). This characterises client-centred occupational therapy intervention and will necessitate client-therapist partnerships in assessment, intervention, and outcome measurement.

Community living poses significant challenges to those who have disabilities. These challenges will be faced most successfully by those people who have been encouraged to assume responsibility for their own well-being, to use their knowledge in a practical way, and to problem solve creatively. At its core, rehabilitation is a learning process. Outcome cannot be measured in terms of a predetermined checklist of skills that have been taught, but rather, by the autonomy and self-determination exhibited by the client (Hammell, 1995b).

ETHICS AND CLIENT-CENTRED INTERVENTION

Ethical decision making in health care consists of the application of theoretical ethics to moral problems. Until recently, the Hippocratic tradition dominated health care, such that patient preferences were set aside if they conflicted with the professional's view of what was in the patient's best interest. Contemporary ethics propose that the competent client is the decision maker, can refuse interventions, and has the right to live at risk. This right may be overruled if the desired intervention is likely to be futile or may be harmful to others (Jonsen, Siegler, & Winslade, 1998). Fundamental to the notion of an autonomy-based ethic is the issue of informed consent. Ethical issues are discussed in Chapter 9. However, it is pertinent to point out that the philosophy of client-centred practice is not unique to occupational therapy, nor is it an optional modus operandi. Rather, current biomedical ethics demand that principles of client autonomy are respected.

I propose that a working knowledge of the principles that inform contemporary biomedical ethics provides a strong endorsement for client-centred practice within occupational therapy and within health care service provision. However, respect for the individual and for client autonomy requires a high standard of information exchange. Occupational therapists have "an ethical and moral responsibility to ensure that clients are as informed as possible of the options and risks associated with possible courses of action" (Health Services Directorate and the Canadian Association of Occupational Therapists, 1993, p. 5).

OUTCOME MEASUREMENT

Demands for accountability are forcing occupational therapists to demonstrate the effectiveness of their interventions. However, some basic questions arise when discussing, using, or reviewing outcome measures. For example, what do the measures contribute to an understanding of the value or success of occupational therapy interventions? What and whose values do the measures represent? To whom do we aim to be accountable? Do the measures reflect outcomes relevant to client goals? Similarly, in long-term studies of client populations, what do the selected outcome measures contribute to enhancing therapists' knowledge of the experience of living with an illness, disadvantage, or disability?

Bauer (1989, p. 199) proposes that rehabilitation services are "an expression of social responsibility towards people who sustain an impairment which results in a temporary or permanent disability."

Outcome measurement must be committed to demonstrating its effectiveness in addressing this responsibility by assessing the consequences, results, and impact of occupational therapy intervention that is based upon the objectives established by the client (Canadian Association of Occupational Therapists, 1991). Occupational therapy intervention is inextricably entwined with assessment, follow-up, and programme evaluation. A philosophical commitment to client-centred practice will, therefore, inform each of these aspects of service delivery and accountability.

Assessment of activities of daily living (ADL)—a euphemism for self-care activities—has been a staple component of occupational therapists' repertoire. However, people with disabilities and, indeed, many therapists have questioned the implicit bias of ADL scales. Scoring systems represent value judgments concerning how an activity should be performed. If a piece of equipment is used to enable a self-care task to be accomplished, for example, a low score is often allocated. Someone with high-lesion quadriplegia, who lives an independent lifestyle by managing and directing others in his or her care, will usually receive no score at all (Law, 1993). For example, the popular Craig Handicap Assessment and Reporting Technique (CHART) (Whiteneck, Charlifue, Gerhart, Overholser, & Richardson, 1992) scores any assistance with self-care activities as indicative of a degree of handicap (low score), yet someone who elects to receive assistance in dressing (for example) may have chosen to conserve time and energy for more productive and personally valuable activities. Whose values are designating this as dependence (Hammell, 1995a)? Further, it is important to consider whether outcome measures reflect client preferences or rather, the traditional value system and role expectations of the dominant culture (Hammell, 1995a). For many people, interdependence may be valued more highly than functional independence.

In an attempt to explore the long-term impact and subjective experience of living with a disability, researchers have begun to use measures of life satisfaction. However, it is evident that even when subjective reports are elicited, these usually constitute subjective assessments of a "researcher-imposed view of life" (Day & Jankey, 1996, p. 46): The people whose lives are being assessed have little or no input into what values should be considered in evaluating their lives. It is not uncommon for a life satisfaction tool developed for use with one population to be used unproblematically with a very different population. In seeking to assess life satisfaction following spinal cord injury, for example, many researchers have used assessment tools borrowed from geriatric literature. Dunnum (1990) used the Life Satisfaction for the Elderly Scale with a group of people who were as young as 18. The Life Satisfaction Index (Neugarten, Havighurst, & Tobin, 1961) was designed to assess quality of life among a healthy, middle-class population in Kansas City.

The amended scale, the LSI-A, was adapted for use in studies of elderly people and is considered to be most suitable for use with people over 65 years of age (Adams, 1969), yet has been used in several studies of young people with spinal cord injuries (Crisp, 1992; Fuhrer, Rintala, Hart, Clearman, & Young, 1992; Rintala, Young, Hart, Clearman, & Fuhrer, 1992). This must be considered in light of evidence that the median age at which spinal cord injury is sustained is 25, with a modal, or most common, age of 19 years (Stover & Fine, 1986). Further, while the majority of seniors are women, about 85% of those with spinal cord injuries are men. The researchers have not articulated their assumption that presumably underpins the use of these assessment tools; that age and gender have no impact upon determinants of life satisfaction or, indeed, that a positive score by a young man on a tool designed for older women produces a meaningful result.

Occupational therapists frequently state that their primary goal is that of enhancing their clients' quality of life. Most commonly, however, outcome measures that have sought to judge the impact and worth of occupational therapy interventions have focused upon functional achievements. Does this reflect a belief that the ability to dress independently, increase the range of motion of a joint or perform bilateral activities, for example, constitutes a form of enhanced quality of life (Hammell, 1995c)? Or is the purpose of judging outcome by measuring specific performance components a means to justify and validate current occupational therapy practice and interventions (Eisenberg & Saltz, 1991)? Most measurement tools assess the ability to perform a task rather than whether that task is actually performed in a real-world context. Weingarden and Martin (1989), for example, found that because of time and energy costs, none of their sample of people with C6 quadriplegia dressed themselves routinely at home, despite being able to do so. This raises an important ethical issue. A successful rehabilitation programme is often considered to be one that demonstrates significant improvement in the level of physical independence attained by clients (Carey, Seibert, & Posavac, 1988; Woolsey, 1985; Yarkony, Roth, Heinemann, & Lovell, 1988). If attention is focused upon teaching skills that are of little or no value to the client (but that reflect favourably upon the service), to whose benefit are these goals being sought (Hammell, 1995a)? Indeed, to whom do we aim to be accountable?

The COPM (Law, Baptiste, Carswell, McColl, Polatajko, & Pollock, 1994) is unique in its client-centred focus and its intent to map the goals and effects of occupational therapy in terms of the client's satisfaction with societal integration, productivity, rewarding leisure pursuits and enlargement of opportunities. The COPM facilitates consideration of the component skills that enable performance of occupations related to self-care, productivity, and leisure, in environmental context. The context or idiosyncratic environmental circumstances will shape the experience of disability or illness and may constitute the locus for intervention. The COPM is a tool that enables the client and therapist to work together to determine goals, define strategies, plan interventions, and assess outcome. It is an important development in providing occupational therapists with a tool to facilitate exploration of the client's biography, life-world, values, and goals: the context for meaningful occupational therapy intervention.

CONCLUSION

Intervention in occupational therapy is the process of interceding to facilitate change in occupational performance. Intervention is one component of the occupational therapy process that cannot be viewed in isolation from assessment, programme planning, follow-up and programme evaluation (Canadian Association of Occupational Therapists, 1991). Client-centred occupational therapy intervention demands an understanding of the meaning of illness or disability within a biography and requires the therapist to work in collaboration with the client to identify goals, plan intervention strategies, measure progress, and assess outcome. The Canadian Association of Occupational Therapists identifies five fundamental elements underpinning occupational therapy intervention: spirituality (concerned with meaning), motivation (inextricably linked to spirituality), the therapeutic relationship as a cornerstone of the client-centred partnership, the teaching-learning process (demonstrated as a bi-directional exchange rather than a uni-directional process), and ethics. These five elements have served also to underpin this chapter. It has been proposed that client-centred occupational therapy intervention is congruent with the ethical principles of autonomy and self-determination. Further, it has been suggested that attempts to recruit client compliance with the goals established for them by their therapists may, at best, be futile. Finally, it has been suggested that, because therapists tend to treat what they assess, assessments and outcome measures should adhere to the principles of client-centred occupational therapy intervention.

REFERENCES

Abberley, P. (1995). Disabling ideology in health and welfare—the case of occupational therapy. *Disabil Society, 10,* 221-232.

Abela, M. B., & Dijkers, M. (1994). Predicting life satisfaction among spinal cord injured patients one to three years post injury (abstract). *Journal of the American Paraplegia Society, 17,* 118.

Adams, D. L. (1969). Analysis of a life satisfaction index. *Journal of Gerontology, 24,* 470-474.

Bauer, D. (1989). *Foundations of physical rehabilitation: a management approach.* Edinburgh: Churchill Livingstone.

Bury, M. (1982). Chronic illness as biographical disruption. *Sociol Health Illn, 4,* 167-182.

Bury, M. (1991). The sociology of chronic illness: a review of research and prospects. *Sociol Health Illn, 13,* 451-468.

Canadian Association of Occupational Therapists (1991). *Occupational therapy guidelines for client-centred practice.* Toronto, ON: Author.

Canadian Association of Occupational Therapists (1997). *Enabling occupation: an occupational therapy perspective.* Ottawa, ON: Author.

Carey, R. G., Seibert, J. H., & Posavac, E. J. (1988). Who makes the most gains in in-patient rehabilitation? An analysis of functional gain. *Archives of Physical Medicine and Rehabilitation, 69,* 337-343.

Chambers Twentieth Century Dictionary (1972). Edinburgh: W&R Chambers Ltd.

Clark, F. A., & Jackson, J. (1989). The application of the occupational science negative heuristic in the treatment of persons with human immunodeficiency infection. *Occupational Therapy Health Care, 6,* 69-91.

Cohen, A. P. (1994). *Self-consciousness. An alternative anthropology of identity.* London: Routledge.

Coles, C. (1989). Self assessment and medical audit: an educational approach. *British Medical Journal, 299,* 807-808.

Cook, D. W. (1981). A multivariate analysis of motivational attributes among spinal cord injured rehabilitation clients. *International Journal of Rehabilitation Research, 4,* 5-15.

Corbin, J., & Strauss, A. L. (1987). Accompaniments of chronic illness: changes in body, self, biography and bio-graphical time. In J. A. Roth & P. Conrad (Eds.). *The experience and management of chronic illness: Research in the sociology of health care,* Vol. 6. Greenwich, CT: JAI Press.

Crepeau, E. B. (1991). Achieving intersubjective understanding: examples from an occupational therapy treatment session. *American Journal of Occupational Therapy, 45,* 1016-1025.

Crisp, R. (1992). The long term adjustment of 60 persons with spinal cord injury. *Aust Psychologist, 27,* 43-47.

Csikszentmihalyi, M. (1993). Activity and happiness: towards a science of occupation. *Occup Science, 1,* 38-42.

Csikszentmihalyi, M., & LeFevre, J. (1989). Optimal experience in work and leisure. *Journal of Personality and Social Psychology, 56,* 815-822.

Curtin, M., & Clarke, H. (1997). Choosing a powered wheelchair: the choice of a client dependent on a ventila-tor. *British Journal of Occupational Therapy, 60,* 156-160.

Curtin, M., & Powell, H. (1997). Responding to individuals in the computer resource room. *British Journal of Occupational Therapy, 60,* 461-462.

Cushman, L. A., & Hassett, J. (1992). Spinal cord injury: 10 and 15 years after. *Paraplegia, 30,* 690-696.

Day, H., & Jankey, S. G. (1996). Lessons from the literature. In R. Renwick, I. Brown, & M. Nagler (Eds.). *Quality of life in health promotion and research.* Thousand Oaks, CA: Sage.

DeVivo, M. J., Black, K. J., Richards, J. S., & Stover, S. L. (1991). Suicide following spinal cord injury. *Paraplegia, 29,* 620-627.

Dunnum, L. (1990). Life satisfaction and spinal cord injury: the patient perspective. *Journal of Neuroscience Nursing, 22,* 43-47.

Eisenberg, M. G., & Saltz, C. C. (1991). Quality of life among aging spinal cord injured persons: long term reha-bilitation outcomes. *Paraplegia, 29,* 514-520.

Entertainment Weekly (1996). A new direction. *Entertainment Weekly, 15 Nov,* 32-37.

Fuhrer, M. J. (1996). The subjective well-being of people with spinal cord injury: relationships to impairment, dis-ability and handicap. *Top SCI Rehabil, 1,* 56-71.

Fuhrer, M. J., Rintala, D. H., Hart, K. A., Clearman, R., & Young, M. E. (1992). Relationship of life satisfaction to impairment, disability and handicap among persons with spinal cord injury living in the community. *Archives of Physical and Medicine and Rehabilitation, 73,* 552-557.

Giddens, A. (1991). *Modernity and self-identity. Self and society in the late modern age.* Stanford, CA: Stanford Uni-versity Press.

Good, B. J. (1994). *Medicine, rationality and experience. An anthropological perspective.* Cambridge: Cambridge University Press.

Hammell, K. W. (1991). *An investigation into the availability and adequacy of social relationships following head injury and spinal cord injury: a study of injured men and their partners.* Unpublished Master of Science disser-tation, Southampton, University of Southampton.

Hammell, K. W. (1992). Psychological and sociological theories concerning adjustment to traumatic spinal cord injury: the implications for rehabilitation. *Paraplegia, 30,* 317-326.

Hammell, K. W. (1994a). Establishing objectives in occupational therapy practice. 1. *British Journal of Occupation-al Therapy, 57,* 9-14.

Hammell, K. W. (1994b). Establishing objectives in occupational therapy practice. 11. *British Journal of Occupa-tional Therapy, 57,* 45-48.

Hammell, K. W. (1994c). Psychosocial outcome following spinal cord injury. *Paraplegia, 32,* 771-779.

Hammell, K. W. (1995a). *Spinal cord injury rehabilitation.* London: Chapman and Hall.

Hammell K. W. (1995b). Application of learning theory in spinal cord injury rehabilitation. Client-centred occupa-tional therapy. *Scandinavian Journal of Occupational Therapy, 2,* 34-39.

Hammell, K. W. (1995c). Quality of life; spinal cord injury; Occupational therapy. Is there a connection? *British Journal of Occupational Therapy, 58,* 151-157.

Hammell, K. W. (1997). *From the neck up: refocusing, doing and becoming following high spinal cord injury (C1-C4): Interview transcripts.* Unpublished.

Hansen, R., & Taylor, J. (1988). *Rick Hansen. Man in motion.* Markham, ON: Penguin Books.

Health Services Directorate and the Canadian Association of Occupational Therapists (1993). *Occupational therapy guidelines for client-centred mental health practice.* Toronto, ON: Canadian Association of Occupational Ther-apists.

Helfrich, C., & Kielhofner, G. (1994). Volitional narratives and the meaning of therapy. *American Journal of Occu-pational Therapy, 48,* 319-326.

Helfrich, C., Kielhofner, G., & Mattingly, C. (1994). Volition as narrative: understanding motivation in chronic illness. *American Journal of Occupational Therapy, 48,* 311-317.

Hooker, E. Z. (1986). Problems of veterans spinal cord injured after age 55: nursing implications. *Journal of Neuroscience Nursing, 18,* 188-195.

Jackson, J. (1995). Sexual orientation: its relevance to occupational science and the practice of occupational therapy. *American Journal of Occupational Therapy, 49,* 669-679.

Jongbloed, L., & Crichton, A. (1990). A new definition of disability: implications for rehabilitation practice and social policy. *Canadian Journal of Occupational Therapy, 57,* 32-38.

Jonsen, A., Siegler, M., & Winslade, W. (1998). *Clinical ethics* (4th ed.). New York: McGraw Hill.

Jordan, S. A., Wellborn, W. R., Kovnik, J., & Saltzstein, R. (1991). Understanding and treating motivational difficulties in ventilator dependent SCI patients. *Paraplegia, 29,* 431-442.

Keith, R. A. (1995). Conceptual basis of outcome measures. *American Journal of Physical Medicine and Rehabilitation, 74,* 73-80.

Kielhofner, G., & Mallinson, T. (1995). Gathering narrative data through interviews: empirical observations and suggested guidelines. *Scandinavian Journal of Occupational Therapy, 2,* 63-68.

Kirchman, M. M. (1986). Measuring the quality of life. *Occupational Therapy Journal of Research, 6,* 21-32.

Kirsh, B. (1996). A narrative approach to addressing spirituality in occupational therapy: exploring personal meaning and purpose. *Canadian Journal of Occupational Therapy, 63,* 55-61.

Kögler, H-H. (1995). The life world. In T. Honderich (Ed.). *The oxford companion to philosophy.* Oxford: Oxford University Press.

Krause, J. S., & Dawis, R. V. (1992). Prediction of life satisfaction after spinal cord injury: A four-year longitudinal approach. *Rehabil Psychol, 37,* 49-60.

Lavine, T. Z. (1984). *From Socrates to Sartre: the philosophic quest.* New York: Bantam.

Law, M. (1991). The environment: a focus for occupational therapy. *Canadian Journal of Occupational Therapy, 58,* 171-180.

Law, M. (1993). Evaluating activities of daily living: directions for the future. *Canadian Journal of Occupational Therapy, 47,* 233-237.

Law, M., Baptiste, S., Carswell, A., McColl, M. A., Polatajko, H., & Pollock, N. (1994). *Canadian occupational performance measure.(2nd ed.)* Toronto, ON: Canadian Association of Occupational Therapists.

Law, M., Steinwender, S., & LeClair, L. (1998). Occupation, health and well-being: a review of research evidence. *Canadian Journal of Occupational Therapy, 65,* 81-91.

Lindberg, M. (1995). Quality of life after subarachnoid haemorrhage, and its relationship to impairments, disabilities and depression. *Scandinavian Journal of Occupational Therapy, 2,* 105-112.

Lorimer, E. A. (1984). Learned helplessness as a framework for practice in long-term care environments. *Aus Occupational Therapy Journal, 31,* 62-67.

Mattingly, C. (1991a). What is clinical reasoning? *American Journal of Occupational Therapy, 45,* 979-986.

Mattingly, C. (1991b). The narrative nature of clinical reasoning. *American Journal of Occupational Therapy, 45,* 998-1005.

Mattingly, C. (1994). The concept of therapeutic 'emplotment.' *Social Science and Medicine, 38,* 811-822.

McColl, M. A., Law, M., & Stewart, D. (1993). *Theoretical basis of occupational therapy.* Thorofare, NJ: SLACK Incorporated.

McKinnon, A. L. (1992). Time use for self care, productivity and leisure among elderly Canadians. *Canadian Journal of Occupational Therapy, 59,* 102-110.

McVeigh, K. (1989). Reflections on the process of education for the patient with high quadriplegia. In G. Whiteneck, C. Adler, R.E. Carter, D.P. Lammertse, S. Manley, R. Menter, K.A. Wagner, C. Wilmot (Eds.). *The management of high quadriplegia: Comprehensive neurologic rehabilitation,* Vol. 1. New York: Demos Publications, pp. 263-270.

Monks, J., & Frankenberg, R. (1995). Being ill and being me: self, body and time in multiple sclerosis narratives. In B. Ingstad & S. R. Whyte (Eds.). *Disability and culture.* Berkeley, CA: University of California Press.

Murphy R. F. (1987). *The body silent.* New York: W. W. Norton.

Neugarten, B. L., Havighurst, R. J., & Tobin, S. S. (1961). The measurement of life satisfaction. *Journal of Gerontology, 16,* 134-143.

Nosek, M., Fuhrer, M. J., & Potter, C. (1995). Life satisfaction of people with physical disabilities: relationship to personal assistance, disability status and handicap. *Rehabil Psychol, 40,* 191-202.

Oliver, M., Zarb, G., Silver, J., Moore, M., & Salisbury, V. (1988). *Walking into darkness. The experience of spinal cord injury.* Basingstoke: Macmillan Press.

Osbon, D. K. (1991). *A Joseph Campbell companion.* New York: Harper Collins.

Oxelgren, C., Harker, J., Hammell, I., & Boyes, B. (1992). *A new beginning. Attendant services through individualised funding.* Regina: South Saskatchewan Independent Living Centre.

Ozer, M. N. (1988). *The management of persons with spinal cord injury.* New York: Demos Publications.

Peloquin, S. M. (1990). The patient-therapist relationship in occupational therapy: understanding visions and images. *American Journal of Occupational Therapy, 44,* 13-21.

Pentland, W., Krupa, T., Lynch, S., & Clark, C. (1992). Community integration for persons with disabilities: working together to make it happen. *Canadian Journal of Occupational Therapy, 59,* 127-130.

Pollock, N. (1993). Client centered assessment. *American Journal of Occupational Therapy, 47,* 298-301.

Rintala, D. H., Young, M. E., Hart, K. A., Clearman, R. R., & Fuhrer, M. J. (1992). Social support and the well being of persons with spinal cord injury living in the community. *Rehabil Psychol, 37,* 155-163.

Robinson, I. (1990). Personal narratives, social careers and medical courses: analyzing life trajectories in autobiographies of people with multiple sclerosis. *Social Science and Medicine, 30,* 1173-1186.

Rogers, J. C., & Figone, J. L. (1980). Traumatic quadriplegia: follow up study of self-care skills. *Archives of Physical Medicine and Rehabilitation, 61,* 316-321.

Rohe, D., & Athelstan, G. T. (1982). Vocational interests of persons with spinal cord injury. *J Counsel Psychol, 29,* 283-291.

Rohe, D. E., & Athelstan, G. T. (1985). Change in vocational interests after spinal cord injury. *Rehabil Psychol, 30,* 131-143.

Schön, D. A. (1983). *The reflective practitioner—how professionals think in action.* San Francisco: Jossey-Bass.

Seligman, M. (1975). *Helplessness: on depression, development and death.* San Francisco: W. H. Freeman and Company.

Siösteen, A., Lundqvist, C., Blomstrand, C., Sullivan, L., & Sullivan, M. (1990). The quality of life of three functional spinal cord injury subgroups in a Swedish community. *Paraplegia, 28,* 476-488.

Strauss, A. L., & Glasser, B. G. (1975). *Chronic illness and the quality of life.* St Louis, MO: Mosby.

Steinglass, P., Temple, S., Lisman, S. A., & Reiss, D. (1982). Coping with spinal cord injury. The family perspective. *General Hospital Psychiatry, 4,* 259-264.

Stover, S. L., & Fine, P. R. (1986). *Spinal cord injury: the facts and figures.* Birmingham, AL: University of Alabama.

Taylor, D. P. (1974). Treatment goals for quadriplegic and paraplegic patients. *American Journal of Occupational Therapists, 28,* 22-29.

Trieschmann, R. B. (1986). The psychosocial adjustment to spinal cord injury. In R. F. Bloch & M. Basbaum (Ed.). *Management of spinal cord injuries.* Baltimore, MD: Williams and Wilkins.

Trieschmann, R. B. (1988). *Spinal cord injuries. Psychological, social and vocational rehabilitation* (2nd ed.). New York: Demos Publications.

Tucker, S. J. (1984). Patient staff interaction with the spinal cord patient. In D. W. Krueger (Ed.). *Rehabilitation psychology.* Rockville, MD: Aspen Publications.

Urbanowski, R., & Vargo, J. (1994). Spirituality, daily practice, and the occupational performance model. *Canadian Journal of Occupational Therapy, 61,* 88-94.

Weingarden, S. I., & Martin, C. (1989). Independent dressing after spinal cord injury: a functional time evaluation. *Archives of Physical Medicine and Rehabilitation, 70,* 518-519.

Whiteneck, G. G., Charlifue, S., Frankel, H., Fraser, M.H., Gardner, B.P., Gerhart, K.A., Krisnan, K.R., Menten, R.R., Nuseibeh, I., Short, D.J. (1992). Mortality, morbidity and psychosocial outcomes of persons spinal cord injured more than 20 years ago. *Paraplegia, 30,* 617-630.

Whiteneck, G. G., Charlifue, S. W., Gerhart, K. A., Overholser, J. D., & Richardson, G. N. (1992). *Guide for use of the CHART: Craig Handicap Assessment and Reporting Technique.* Englewood, CO: Craig Hospital.

Wilcock, A. A. (1993). Editorial. *Occupational Science, 1,* 1-2.

Williams, G. H. (1987). Disablement and the social context of daily activity. *Int Disabil Studies, 9,* 97-102.

Woolsey, R. M. (1985). Rehabilitation outcome following spinal cord injury. *Archives of Neurology, 42,* 116-119.

Yarkony, G. M., Roth, E. J., Heinemann, A. W., & Lovell, L. (1988). Rehabilitation outcomes in C6 tetraplegia. *Paraplegia, 26,* 177 185.

Yerxa, E. J., & Baum, S. (1986). Engagement in daily occupations and life satisfaction among people with spinal cord injuries. *Occupational Therapy Journal of Research, 6,* 271-283.

Yerxa, E. J., & Locker, S. B. (1990). Quality of time use by adults with spinal cord injuries. *American Journal of Occupational Therapy, 44,* 318-326.

CLIENT-CENTRED OCCUPATIONAL THERAPY: ETHICS AND IDENTITY

SARAH ROCHON, MSc(T), OT(C), SUE BAPTISTE, MHSc, OT(C)

INTRODUCTION

"Ethics is broadly concerned with how persons ... act, or should act, in relations with others" (Hall, 1993, p. 3). By definition, it suggests rules that govern relationships and cooperation within society. Ethical behaviour can be complex. Within a practice profession, in the simplest terms, ethics presumes the disposition to act in a way that offers good and no harm to one's clients. More complex principles include "informed consent, paternalistic deception, and privileged confidentiality," which are common concepts undertaken in applied ethics courses within the professions (Rest, 1994, p. 9). Codes of ethics within professions require professionals to put clients' interests or interests of the group to which they belong ahead of their own (Pavelko, 1972).

Becoming ethically sensitive to support a client-centred process of practice requires a level of sophistication in professional identity beyond the usual expectations of professional codes of conduct. It requires a fundamental shift in identity moving the occupational therapist from the role of expert advisor to that of partner and facilitator with expertise (Figure 9-1).

On the surface, a decision to practice in a client-centred fashion poses little or no dilemma given the current 1990s social context. At a sub-societal level, it is supported by what Rest (1994) refers to as "Western Liberalism": the rational choice to value individuals and their rights within society as a valuable consumer. Brockett (1993) endorses this view of valuing the individual as a force in support of client-centred practice within occupational therapy. She further suggests that another driving societal influence is of a socio-political nature. The forces in support of health promotion are derived both from a consumer movement, but also from a governmental and insurer's need to relinquish societal responsibility for health back to the individual, thereby cutting costs and reducing deficits associated with the ongoing health care industry.

Whatever the source of motivation, the desirability of practising in a client-centred fashion is clearly evident in current health care and occupational therapy practice. Despite this apparent social sanction, there are existing tensions that must be overcome if therapists are to be able to practice in a client-centred fashion. Brockett (1993) postulated that the "call to" or vocation to help another person can be antithetical to the Kantian phi-

```
┌─────────────────────────────────────────────────────────────┐
│                                                             │
│        FROM ──────────────────────────────► TO             │
│        expert advisor                partner with expertise │
│                                                             │
└─────────────────────────────────────────────────────────────┘
```

Figure 9-1. Fundamental Shift in Professional Identity.

losophy needed to allow one's client to be a self-determining individual. Freire (1992) has suggested that

> "*Any situation in which 'a' objectively exploits 'b' or hinders [b]'s pursuit of self-affirmation as a responsible person is one of oppression. Such a situation in itself constitutes violence, even when sweetened by false generosity because it interferes with man's ontological and historical vocation to be more fully human.*" (Freire, 1992, p. 40)

In order to avoid the pitfall of applying caring as a form of social control, the practitioner must cultivate an advanced awareness of the circumstances in which his or her values, duties, rights, and principles or needs are in conflict with those of the client and his or her chosen life course. Such awareness is cultivated through personal reflection, including the clarification of one's values and the development of rational ethical principles that can serve as resources in times of crisis and self-doubt (Gellerman, Frankel, & Randenson, 1990).

This chapter presents central and key dispositions essential for the occupational therapist to adopt in the promotion of a client-centred practice. The reader is challenged to review his or her own attitudes, values, and practices in considering these various key concepts. The issues discussed in the chapter are not all-inclusive but will provoke the kind of self-reflective inquiry that can set a practitioner on the road to client-centred practice.

In order to begin this journey, it is essential to contemplate what it means to be human and what motivates human beings to think, develop values and principles, and act according to a sense of right and wrong. An additional area of importance for reflection and the establishment of a comfort zone is that of professional identity. Thus, a detailed discussion of this component of ethical practice will be shared, together with self-reflective exercises intended to assist the therapist in gaining a sense of self; a sense of self that will enable the therapist to translate personal values and beliefs into operational behaviours.

THERAPIST'S VIEW OF HUMANS AND HUMAN MOTIVATION

The *Canadian Occupational Therapy Guidelines for Client-Centred Practice* define motivation as "the dynamic or inner force that brings a person to act according to a sense of purpose and direction in life" (Canadian Association of Occupational Therapists, 1991, p. 59). This view mandates that the therapist regard humans as fully capable of choice, adopting a perspective that behaviour is adaptable and changeable based upon cognitive decisions made by each person. This disposition calls to mind the work of Weiner (1992), who suggested that theories in motivation cluster into one of two categories.

He contends that the early dominant metaphor for motivation in the first half of the 20th century was that man operated like a machine. He argues that the emerging theories of motivation give increasing credit to the constructs of personal choice and self-determination in shaping behaviour. As Descartes stated: "I think, therefore, I am" (Weiner, 1992, p. 153).

The history of theory development for occupational therapy indicates an early tendency to borrow and adapt theoretical traditions of other fields (psychology, psychiatry, sociology, etc.). This was a dominant practice until the mid to late 1970s (Kielhofner, 1983; McColl, Law & Stewart, 1993). The dominant schools within psychology and motivation in the early half of the century were psychoanalytic theory, behaviourism, and development (McColl, Law, & Stewart, 1993). All three of these perspectives assume the human is motivated by sources other than personal choice: needs and drives, the reinforcements and contingencies of learning and the environment, and sequential maturational, innate developmental milestones, respectively (McColl, Law, & Stewart, 1993; Reed, 1984). These three dominant traditions are identified by Weiner (1992) as the metaphor of human as machine, driven by external or pre-programmed forces.

In the past two decades, we have seen significant development in theory within occupational therapy, led by scholars within the field. Key works have embraced the notion of human volition and personal choice as a powerful motivator for adaptation and change (Christianson & Baum, 1997; McColl, Law, & Stewart, 1993; Kielhofner, 1987). The embracing of theory developed by profession-specific scholars has been cited as evidence of maturation within the field (McColl, Law, & Stewart, 1993; Kielhofner, 1983).

This brief contextual overview of theories of motivation within occupational therapy suggests two issues for the therapist as he or she adopts a client-centred practice. Firstly, the combined notion of era of graduation from occupational therapy education and currency of theoretical assumptions suggest that those therapists who cling to theoretical notions that postulate the individual is controlled by external means, or what Weiner (1992) has suggested as machine-like metaphors, will have difficulty adopting this form of practice. This hypothesis was demonstrated in a small study involving therapists' adoption of a client-centred form of practice (Rochon, 1994). In this study, the therapist who most heartedly rejected a client-centred process of care presented the following metaphor for her practice:

> "For me, practising occupational therapy is rather like being an architect. As I see it, someone approaches the architect with a need or an idea. It is the job of the architect to draw up some plans and designs that will take into consideration the need or idea of the person, whether or not it is feasible, as well as the resources available. As the building is under construction, the architect gives continual direction and feedback... Of course, as obstacles are met along the way, the architect may need to modify and adapt his plans. Finally, the architect stands back to look at the building that is in place, acknowledging that he had a hand in the fashioning of it. However, it may be frustrating if it is not possible because the builders are on strike!" (Rochon, 1994, p. 110)

In analysing this metaphor, the respondent clearly stated that she believed that she was the driving force in intervention, stating, "I design a treatment plan based upon the client's needs, taking into account whether the goals of the client are realistic, as well as resources available. I communicate regularly with clients at all stages of treatment. I direct clients in using various skills and to utilise available resources. I assist clients in problem solving" (Rochon, 1994, p. 110).

Beyond the personal history of the therapist and his or her development and personal biases related to theory, the history of the profession of occupational therapy and where it currently stands in relation to the development of theory is also significant in terms of readiness to adopt a client-centred approach to care. As a practice profession, we must constantly be aware of the emerging development of knowledge within other compatible fields. Clearly, if we value a client-centred approach, we must choose those theories that view humans in a compatible vein.

THERAPISTS' PROFESSIONAL IDENTITY

"... What is requisite, if I am to be treating you as the person you are, is that I find out what your self-conception is, and respond to that rather than paying attention to characteristics of yours which are not something you take to be important to the person you are." (Spelman, 1977, p. 152)

Like any component of self-concept, professional identity is an individual, ever-changing, ephemeral personal construct. Out of respect for this reality, this section takes a personal, self-reflective approach. The first two parts of this chapter presented information; this piece, however, presents challenges for the reader. It outlines six exercises that, if followed, will guide the reader in a self-reflective analysis of his or her current professional identity and readiness to engage in a client-centred process and partnership to facilitate an optimal delivery of care through ethical facilitation. These exercises prompt consideration of professional attitudes, commitment, and mission for practice. The process will require the collection of data over a 1- to 2-week time period. Review of the data will follow at a later time to allow for distancing from the data collection itself. Keeping a journal to capture one's reactions and insights is recommended.

Table 9-1 outlines each of the five exercises, identifies the name for the process and the theoretical base of each, as well as provides key sources or originating authors.

In order to become comfortable with one's ethical grounding, which, in turn, results from a combination of values, beliefs, learned behaviours, and personality preferences, it is essential that the individual therapist embrace an open approach to self-exploration and a willingness to review, examine, and change. Engaging in the exercises interspersed throughout the chapter will prompt the discovery of personal role parameters and elements of satisfaction and professional meaning that drive the manner in which client/therapist relationships are created and nurtured.

	Table 9-1	
Exercise	**Theoretical Base Title for the Process**	**Source(s)**
#1	occupational therapy theory transformative learning activity configuration reflective journalling human/organization development personal mission	Moorehead, 1969 Bridges, 1991 Brookfield, 1987 Mezirow, 1990 Rochon & Worth, 1995 Covcy, 1989 Rochon 1993
#2	adult development adult learning theory life-line review	Sugarman, 1986 Spencer [ICA], 1989 Rochon 1993
#3	human/organization development exposing the left-hand or "X/Y case"	Argyris & Schon, 1974 Argyris et al., 1985 Rochon, 1994 Rochon & Worth, 1995 Cranton, 1992 Cranton, 1995
#4	transformative learning metaphor analysis	Candy, 1986 Hunt, 1988 Hunt & Gow, 1984 Rochon, 1994 Cranton, 1995
#5	personal construct theory repertory grid	Kelly, 1995, 1963 Hunt, 1988 Hunt & Gow, 1984 Rochon, 1994 Rest & Narvaez, 1994
#6	calls for a summary of findings of the other exercises	

Exercise 1. Personal Mission Versus the Realities of Practice

I.   In your journal, write a paragraph describing why you chose to be an occupational therapist, and set it aside.

II.   Consider the quote:

 In medical culture, occupational therapists are often seen as technicians, or even playladies, who occupy patients hospital time with checker games and craft groups. From a biomedical perspective, chronic illness and disability are physiological problems. But from an occupational therapy perspective, disability is not only an injury to the body, it is an injury to the patient s life. Occupational therapists have the task of helping the handicapped become more functionally independent . This can be treated as a technical task, one of helping clients improve their motor skills and learn to use special adaptive equipment. Or it can be treated as addressing the profound difficulty of how disabled persons are going to be able to continue to live meaningful lives burdened with bodies [and minds] that no longer allow them to carry out those occupations that gave their lives meaning and purpose, which in turn gave them a sense of self. (Mattingly, 1991, p. 254-255)

III. Jot down in your journal any reactions you have to Mattingly s description of the realities of practicing as an occupational therapist.

IV. Spend the next week keeping a log of the activities in which you engage professionally, a tool which is well known to occupational therapists. Now you will apply it to yourself! Make a schedule for one week s work; note in point form or short sentences what you were actually doing at each time on the schedule.

Table 9-2 provides a brief example.

Table 9-2

		Mon	Tues	Wed	Thurs	Fri
0830	Attended rounds haemotology unit					
0930	Made splint Mrs. X					
1030	Consulted re: Mrs. Y and discharged her home					
1130						
1230						
Etc.						

At the end of the week, review the log and make a list of the verbs you used. For example, in Table 9-2 the verbs include attended and consulted. Review what you have written in your journal and place the verb list next to Mattingly s (1991) quote, and use these insights to help you write a paragraph in response to each of the following statements:

My mission in being an occupational therapist is...

In reality, my practice is...

PROFESSIONALISM

For the purposes of this discussion, professionalism is defined as the manner in which a practitioner interprets and enacts the mantle of being a professional. The hallmark of being a professional is the possession of a unique body of knowledge (Purtilo, 1990). Indeed, Purtilo (1990) contends that there is only one distinguishing feature between the professional and the client as they embark upon a helping relationship and that is the unique knowledge base held only by the professional. The professional brings expertise, and the client is in need of that specialised knowledge (Pavelko, 1972).

The codes of ethics for professional groups hold key universal commonalities. These include a mandate that the professional must at all times put the client's needs above his or her own; a requirement to maintain currency of professional knowledge and skill; and strictures to safeguard the confidentiality of client information (Canadian Association of Occupational Therapists, 1996). These codes ensure that a client/consumer can expect to receive an appropriate level of expertise when entering into a relationship with a professional. They do not, however, ensure that the professional will function in any particular mode of partnership with that client. The decision to function in a client-centred fashion involves a moral choice that remains with each individual therapist. This decision is inextricably linked to the therapist's interpretation of what it means to be a professional. The previous section challenged readers to consider what being an occupational therapist means to them and their identities. This section addresses factors that can shape a practitioner's interpretation of what it means to be a professional within a rehabilitation context. A multitude of factors can serve to shape the way in which a practitioner enacts his or her own professionalism. In assisting the reader to consider the moral decision of whether to embark upon a client-centred process of practice, three of these factors are discussed:

- the practitioner's preferred style of interacting and sharing expertise
- his or her belief regarding most appropriate service
- the manner in which problems are framed and set the context for clinical reasoning

Exercise 2. Career Review

I.   Draw a time line for your career in the service and support of clients, marking off at intervals of two to three years.

Table 9-3 represents an example.

Table 9-3

CAREER:	1976*	1979**	1982	1985	1988	Etc.

*1976: graduation; hired at first job; made group therapy coordinator on unit; excellent progress with client X; difficulty in team re: role

**1979: suicide of client Y; began working with community outreach clinic

Etc.

II. In the time line, cite any highs and lows in your career accomplishments (see Table 9-3).

III. In your journal, write two paragraphs:

The common themes in the high points of my career are...

The common themes in the low points of my career are...

Contrast the following metaphor with the one presented earlier in this chapter. Both therapists work with the same clientele: adults with significant mental illnesses.

For me, practising occupational therapy is like being a coach for the sport, sailboarding. We begin the process with discussions out-of-context, sharing key tips and learning principles that will guide the process. The real work begins when we are both in the water together. The client or student is still able to ask questions: e.g. how to address the board? What really are the wind conditions today? How choppy is the surface of the water? I still have time to review the learner s readiness and to offer some last minute tips. But before long, the person has hopped on the board and is beginning to drift away. He must now find his own balance, begin to read the wind and start to manoeuvre around the board in a way that will set things in motion. The more he attempts to gain his own control, the farther he drifts away. I am left on shore, calling tips and directions from the side, but ultimately, he is in charge. Before long a gust of wind sweeps him away and I watch him as he attempts to manoeuvre across the lake. I remain up to my knees in water communicating with hand signals and short curt tips that can be heard

---

Exercise 3. Taking a Look Back

I.   Pick one high point and one low point from your career review.

II. For each incident, set up two blank columns as in Table 9-4. On the right hand column of each page, describe your recollection of the selected past experience. On the left hand column, write your answer to questions pertaining to the experience.

Table 9-4

	1. Describe the actual experience: a) high or b) low.
2. What were you thinking, doing, feeling at the time?	
3. What do you think your colleagues or clients were thinking, feeling, doing at the time?	
4. What does this tell you about your conception of success in your career?	
5. What does it tell you about your beliefs about failure in your career?	
6. How would your colleagues or clients appraise your success or failure?	

---

on the water. At some point, he wends his way back close, and now in ear shot, seeking advice on how to improve his skill or deal with an unexpected challenge. Before long, he is skittering away, caught by another gust of wind, and enjoying his new-found abilities. I take my joy in the hopeful fact that my involvement has helped him to learn this sport in a safe, efficient and less daunting manner. (Rochon & Worth, 1995)

The two metaphors: occupational therapist as architect and occupational therapist as coach are remarkably distinct. The architect image conveys a view of expertise as being a valuable commodity that must be apportioned in accordance with the wisdom of the expert. The coach scenario suggests that the client controls the need for expertise and that the coach is responsible for providing that expertise when requested. The former view of expertise as a commodity to be apportioned is similar to what Freire (1992) refers to as the banking concept of education. In reviewing the practice of teaching, he has said:

Knowledge is a gift bestowed by those who consider themselves knowledgeable upon those who may [be considered] to know nothing. Projecting an absolute ignorance onto others, a characteristic of the ideology of oppression, negates education and knowledge as processes of inquiry. The teacher presents himself to his students as their necessary opposite, by considering their ignorance absolute, he justifies his own existence. (Freire, 1992, p. 58)

Freire s appraisal could fit for the architect-like therapist. This, however, may be a harsh judgment. Perhaps that first architect-like therapist is unable to consider the possibility that the practice of occupational therapy merely improves the process of recovery rather than being the essential cause for success in rehabilitation. The coach-like therapist appears to hold this perspective and to have reconciled her role as one who can make the process better. She appears to accept that recovery occurs because of the strength, will, and power of the individual client. She hopes that her intervention will make the process easier, safer, and less traumatic.

Service is portrayed very differently in each scenario. The architect scenario suggests that service is the drawing together of knowledge to create a design. The product of that service is the intervention plan. The job is complete when the design is perfected. Service within the coaching story appears as a readiness to help. Expertise is what is drawn from the therapist, based upon the requests and needs of the client. This situation implies that the nature of the expertise shared, while following common principles, is necessarily individualised. Just what a particular client will need is somewhat unpredictable and, in some ways, haphazard, as is the wind that catches the sailboard s sail. The differences in the views of power and accountable practice within these two metaphors are important. The architect holds herself separate from the client, embroidering her talent and personality upon the plan. The coach jumps into the water with the client, partnering to share her expertise and becoming accountable within that partnership for the progress that the client is able to make.

Exercise 4. Metaphor for Practice

I.   At two points in this chapter, therapists own metaphors for practice are shared. Refer to these examples and write a metaphor for *your* practice, beginning with the statement:

For me, practising occupational therapy is like...

II.   When you have written a metaphor with which you are satisfied, that really rings true for you, use your journal to comment upon the following:

- What makes the metaphor ring true for you?
- Describe how well it reflects the complexity, breadth and depth of your practice.
- How does it portray the way you relate to clients and how clients relate to you?
- What does it say about how you derive meaning from your work?

The professionalism of any therapist occurs in a context. That social context influences the therapist s ability to practice in concert with his or her beliefs. The biomedical culture sees diagnosis and the ensuing problem lists as the appropriate frame upon which to design service. Such a framework is an uneasy fit for the therapist whose business is helping people to become more functionally independent and resume a meaningful existence. This tension between the beliefs of occupational therapists and the beliefs of the dominant health care culture has been documented by many writers (Yerxa, 1983, 1992; Maxwell & Maxwell, 1980; Mattingly & Fleming, 1994; Fleming, 1991a). Mattingly (1991a) and Mattingly & Fleming (1994), in their studies of the clinical reasoning of occupational therapists, have eloquently captured many of the strategies therapists use to reconcile this tension in beliefs.

One of the most common strategies used by therapists appears to be the incorporation of the biomedical diagnosis or problem list as the beginning point for therapy. Once therapy has begun, however, these reference points lose their importance, being relinquished for more salient analyses of the person's motivation, goals for life, standards for quality of living, and readiness for learning and enhancement of ability (Mattingly & Fleming, 1994; Fleming, 1991a, 1991b). For example, the bio-psycho-social framework has been a dominant perspective for identifying and organizing treatment of problems within the biomedical sphere for the past 25 years. This system supports the development of an intervention plan by building a framework that lists key problems for the client (Engel, 1977). Occupational therapists have incorporated that perspective into their practice, but, in recognising the limitations of a singular view on problems, have extended and adapted it to their own use. This perspective has been called the rehabilitation approach (McColl, Law, & Stewart, 1993). In the rehabilitation approach, therapists also document under the same three categories—bio-psycho-social—the assets that the client brings to managing his or her life problems. This balance of information allows the therapist to see a picture that more truly reflects an understanding of the person within their total life context. Such a method of "framing" problems appears to reconcile the need for common language with the biomedical health care team and the occupational therapist's own need for a perspective on occupational function (Rochon, 1993). It allows therapists, within the context of their work, to report in language that is compatible with a dominant culture and, at the same time, consider issues of importance within their professional practice and view of their own professionalism.

Within occupational therapy, a tool has been developed to ensure that a therapist uses a client-centred approach in planning and evaluating the outcomes of treatment. This tool, the Canadian Occupational Performance Measure (Law, Baptiste, Carswell-Opzoomer, McColl, Polatajko & Pollock, 1994), uses early information about clients' own goals in the context of self-care, productivity, and leisure, for the guiding framework for therapy (see Chapter 5). It has been recognized as a key enabler to both therapists and their clients in moving toward client-centred practice (Rochon, 1994). This tool, however, reframes the language in which the therapist presents client goals and, ultimately, the plans and outcome of their interventions. This application of language compatible with the fundamental beliefs of occupational therapy can prove to be a barrier between the therapist and the health care team upon which he or she works, as illustrated in the following quote:

"... on one of the task forces that I'm on to look at program development, I've noticed that I often will say—it's really important that whatever we do, that we set up with the person's goals in mind. What I'm realising is that my definition of goals is quite different from the treatment team's. [For example], I'd say, I'd like to see team meetings run based on the patient's goals and just have those goals focused on within the team meeting, and, I'd like to see charting set up with the goals in mind. But Nursing seem to have their own system and it's their own opinion of what's going on vs. having the person state what they feel that is their problem. So whenever I mention it, it's kind of—yeah, okay—it's always side-stepped. Then I feel that I really want to push that a little bit more. That we should have their goals set up, but we should have them doing the setting up. They'll [referring to the health care team members] have their own view and will say—these are the patient's goals, but it's their goals as opposed to the patient's own goals." (Rochon, 1994, p. 98)

This disparate view and the social press for conforming to it, implied in the workplace, was cited as the reason for this therapist choosing to seek employment at a more client-centred health-care organization. This individual's experience suggests that any therapist's enactment of his or her own professionalism and the associated moral decisions he or she makes are highly influenced by the dominant culture in which practice occurs. The decision to adopt client-centred practice and the sense of power to do so can be strongly enhanced or undermined by circumstances outside the individual therapist's control and, therefore, inherently involves risks to be weighed and overcome.

CULTURE AS AN ELEMENT OF ETHICAL PRACTICE

As the underpinnings of occupational therapy practice are being explored and more clearly articulated, one major area for awareness and sensitive attention is emerging; namely, the cultural environment of clients, be the client an individual, a family system or sub-system, or a social institution, such as industry or business (Baptiste, 1988). Any discussion of client-centred practice would be radically incomplete without addressing the multiple faces of cultural environments that impact directly on the establishment of facilitative client/therapist partnerships. "Culture" has many differing meanings and interpretations, but for the purposes of this current discussion, the term "culture" will be seen to encompass ethnicity, formal belief systems, organisational environments, and professional orientation.

Canada, the United States, and other countries possess rich tapestries of many cultures, which have immediate and obvious impact on the building of therapeutic relationships with clients. However, one of the least recognised is that of the health care process itself. Few, if any, health care practitioners are actively aware that they bring a firmly established culture and language to the therapeutic interface. When we speak of "completing an assessment" or developing a "care management plan," there are few clients who understand enough of this language to provide them with adequate comfort to move forward with the therapist with an attitude of trust, openness, and sharing. All of these

Exercise 5. Comparing Styles of Cooperation

I.   Begin this exercise by writing each of the following statements on an index card or piece of paper. You will have six cards.

- Card # 1: Prefers to promote cooperation by ensuring that all parties are clear about what is expected of them.

- Card # 2: Likes to promote cooperation by finding a way to make a deal.

- Card # 3: Believes that if you treat everyone kindly that cooperation will naturally follow.

- Card # 4: Prefers to use rules, policies, etc. as a way of promoting cooperation.

- Card # 5: Likes to promote cooperation by developing consensus and bringing everyone on board to follow the wishes of the group.

- Card # 6: Likes to promote cooperation by engaging people with an impartial view and equipping them to apply a rational process.

II.   Use these statement cards to compare your own most preferred way of achieving cooperation with that of the environment (team, organisation, etc.) within which you work. You will compare the statements in groups of three (triads) choosing the two that are closest to the truth, either for you or your organisation.

III.   Record your responses on charts similar to Tables 9-5a and 9-5b.

Table 9-5a

Combination to be compared	Pairs of statements closest to how I like to promote cooperation
(e.g) 2, 3, & 6	_____ + _____
5, 6, & 1	_____ + _____

Table 9-5b

Combination to be compared	Pairs of statements closest to how I like to promote cooperation
(e.g) 3, 4, & 5	_____ + _____
6, 1, & 2	_____ + _____

IV.   Using the statement cards, review any pattern that emerges.

V.   In your log, write three paragraphs by completing the following statements:

I like to promote cooperation by...

My workplace appears to like to promote cooperation by...

These two situations...

attributes are central to the concept of client-centredness, and, hence, if these are not present, the task of creating a true partnership becomes increasingly difficult.

Similarly, all clients arrive with their own assumptions based on social and cultural training throughout the life span, tempered by previous experiences. Many clients who come from ethnic backgrounds that are diverse from those that dominate North American society approach an interview with the therapist with expectations or fears. These fears may not be minimised, depending on the approach taken, in turn, by the therapist. Many clients "bring with them beliefs about what causes symptoms—everything from the 'evil eye' to 'too much bile gone to the head' to 'germs'—and about suitable treatments, ranging from talismans to aspirin to coriander tea" (Waxler-Morrison, Anderson, & Richardson, 1990). For example, Canada is populated largely by diverse immigrant groups, and, thus, there are additional concerns relative to the nature and status of being an "immigrant." Most immigrant groups share three common bonds when attempting to integrate into their new life: lack of facility with the language, minimal financial and social resources, and a confusion and fear of the unknown bureaucracies that surround them. When attempting then to create a climate of security and equality within the therapeutic partnership, it is essential to consider these basic inadequacies (Waxler-Morrison, Anderson, & Richardson, 1990). Consideration must be given to the facilitation of the interview/intervention environment through consideration of language and terminology used, the utilization of the services of an interpreter when appropriate, and the consideration of involving family or social network members to ease the transition. Similarly, consideration relative to the careful use of financial resources coupled with an explanation of support available is critically important. When it comes to explaining the vagaries and complexities of the health care systems themselves, time spent in minute detail and repetition is never wasted.

Unfortunately, together with these shared areas of concern, there exists within immigrant populations a shared social position of minimal power.

"Although cultural minority groups do hold distinct beliefs about 'right' behaviour and values, and about appropriate responses to misbehaviour, they are often less well-off and have less political power than the majority. Therefore, minority culture often implies both distinctive cultural beliefs and less powerful social positions. Both characteristics are reflected in the problems these sub-groups and health professional have in devising mutually satisfactory health care." (Waxler-Morrison, Anderson, & Richardson, 1990 p. 9-10)

Other areas for attention, when seeking to gain sensitivity to cultural differences, include disparities in the understanding and acceptance of space, time, nonverbal communication, and role expectations (Purtillo, 1990). Many professional dilemmas emerge from consideration of these additional issues. Risks may appear to be inherent in moving forward in directions identified by the client; however, it is incumbent upon the therapist to determine whether his or her definition of 'risk' stems from 'true' risk to the client or from a cultural or values-based differential. For example, the client with chronic back pain who has led a highly physical lifestyle may consider getting back on water skis to be a low risk activity, considering his or her true wish to return to skydiving. The therapist may have to struggle with his or her own sense of safety and must reframe his or her input to his or her client through the client s eyes, providing this client with key information about body mechanics and supportive harnesses that can serve to minimize the risk. Similarly, client expectations of the role of the therapist may lead to a disparity between what is deemed to be competent practice and what is experienced through the therapeutic interactions. A client may view expertise as a state of knowing and then of telling rather than advising and guiding. If the client s needs are not met within the context of facilitation, this may result in the client choosing to refuse treatment. Again, it becomes the therapist s responsibility to explain and explore the interface of roles in order to allow the relationship to flourish. Despite all best efforts, a positive outcome is not always possible, and the termination of a therapeutic partnership should be seen as inevitable from time to time.

When addressing the relationship between cultural elements of the therapist/client relationship and the mission of ethical practice, there are multiple issues of which to be aware, from both the perspective of the client and that of the therapist. In essence, the hub of need centres around an honest willingness to listen to the client; to read between the lines; not to take communication (or lack of it) purely at face value; to eagerly explore the cultural complexities that potentially are present at any client/therapist interaction; to guard against assumptions. With this approach to practice, there will be minimal risk of the partners diverging along totally different pathways, but, instead, converging with mutual understanding and shared goals and outcomes.

SUMMARY

This chapter has presented some of the many faces of client-centred practice in an ethical context. The reader is encouraged to engage in a process of personal reflection to develop, internalise, and own a truly ethical practice style. There is sincere recognition of the difficulties inherent in this process, but, to be authentically client-centred, this exploration is paramount.

Exercise 6. Drawing Your Own Conclusions

I.   In your journal, write one page describing key elements of your professional identity revealed in the previous five exercises.

II.   Review that description, being critical about your comfort and readiness to engage in a client-centred approach to your practice.

REFERENCES

Argyris, C., & Schon, D. (1974). *Theory in practice: Increasing professional effectiveness.* San Francisco: Jossey-Bass Publishers.

Argyris, C., Putnam, R., & McLain Smith, D. (1985). *Action science: Concepts, methods and skills for research and intervention.* San Francisco: Jossey-Bass Publishers.

Baptiste, S. (1988). Culture, activity and chronic pain. Muriel Driver Lecture. *Canadian Journal of Occupational Therapy, 55,* 179-184.

Bridges, W. (1991). *Managing transitions: Making the most of change.* Reading, MA: Addison-Wesley Publishing Co.

Brockett, M. (1993). *An ethic of respect for client-centred partnerships.* Unpublished EdD Thesis, Toronto, ON: Ontario Institute for Studies in Education, University of Toronto.

Brookfield, S. D. (1987). *Developing critical thinkers: Challenging adults to explore alternative ways of thinking.* San Francisco: Jossey-Bass Publishers.

Canadian Association of Occupational Therapists. (1991). *Occupational therapy guidelines for client- centred practice.* Toronto, ON: CAOT Publication ACE.

Canadian Association of Occupational Therapists. (1996). *Code of ethics.* Ottawa, ON: CAOT.

Candy, P. C. (1986). The eye of the beholder: Metaphor in adult education research. *International Journal of Life Long Learning, 5*(2), 87-111.

Christensen, C., & Baum, C. (1997). *Occupational therapy: Enabling function and well-being* (2nd ed.). Thorofare, NJ: SLACK Incorporated.

Covey, S. (1989) *The seven habits of highly effective people: Restoring the character ethic.* New York: Fireside Books, Simon & Shuster.

Cranton, P. (1992). *Working with adult learners.* Toronto, ON: Wall & Emerson, Inc.

Cranton, P. (1995). *Understanding and promoting transformational learning: A guide for educators of adults.* San Francisco: Jossey-Bass Publishers.

Engel, G. (1977). The need for a new medical model: a challenge for biomedicine. *Science, 196,* 129-136.

Fleming, M. H. (1991a). Clinical reasoning in medicine compared with clinical reasoning in occupational therapy. *American Journal of Occupational Therapy, 45*(11), 988-997.

Fleming, M. H. (1991b). The therapist with the three-track mind. *American Journal of Occupational Therapy, 45*(11), 1007-1015.

Freire, P. (1992). *Pedagogy of the oppressed.* New York: The Continuum Publishing Co.

Gellermann, W., Frankel, M.S., & Ladenson, R.F. (1990). *Values and ethics in human systems development: responding to dilemmas in professional life.* San Francisco: Jossey-Bass Publishers.

Hall, W. D. (1993). *Making the right decision: Ethics for managers.* New York: John Wiley & Sons, Inc.

Hunt, D. (1988). *Beginning with ourselves: In practice, theory and human affairs.* Cambridge, MA: Brookline Books.

Hunt, D. E., & Gow, J. (1984). How to be your own best theorist II. *Theory into Practice, 18,* 64-71.

Kelly, G. (1995). *The psychology of personal constructs.* (2 volumes). New York: W. W. Norton & Co.

Kelly, G. (1963). *Theory of personality: The psychology of personal constructs.* New York: W. W. Norton & Co.

Kielhofner, G. (Ed.) (1983). *Health through occupation: Theory and practice in occupational therapy.* Philadelphia: F. A. Davis Co.

Law, M., Baptiste, S., Carswell, A., McColl, M. A., Polatajko, H., & Pollock, N. (1994). *Canadian Occupational Performance Measure.* (2nd ed). Toronto, ON: Canadian Association of Occupational Therapists.

Mattingly, C. (1991). Narrative reflections on practical actions: Learning experiments in reflective storytelling. In D. A. Schon (Ed.), *The reflective turn: Case studies in and on educational practice.* New York: Teachers' College Press, pp. 235-282.

Mattingly, C., & Fleming, M. H. (1994). *Clinical reasoning: Forms of inquiry in therapeutic practice.* Philadelphia: F. A. Davis Company.

Maxwell, J. D., & Maxwell, M. P. (1980). Inner fraternity and outer sorority: Social structure and the professionalization of occupational therapy. In A. Wipper (Ed.). *Essays in honour of Oswald Hall.* [Carlton Library Series]. Ottawa, ON: MacMillan, pp. 330-358.

McColl, M. A., Law, M., & Stewart, D. (1993). *The theoretical foundations of occupation: An annotated bibliography of occupational therapy in the 20th century in North America.* Thorofare, NJ: SLACK Incorporated.

Mezirow, J. (1990). *Fostering critical reflection in adulthood*. San Francisco: Jossey-Bass Publishers.

Moorehead, M. L. (1969). The occupational history. *American Journal of Occupational Therapy, 23,* 329-334.

Pavelko, R. (1972). *Sociological perspectives on occupations*. Itasca, IL: Peacock Publishers.

Purtilo, R. (1990). *Health professional and patient interaction*. Toronto, ON: W. B. Saunders Company.

Reed, K. L. (1984). *Models of practice in occupational therapy*. Baltimore: Williams & Wilkins.

Rest, J. R. (1994). Background: Theory and Research. In J. R. Rest & D. Narvaez (Eds.). *Moral development in the professions: Psychology and applied ethics*. Hillsdale, NJ: Lawrence Erlbaum Associates, Publishers.

Rest, J. R., & Narvaez, D. (Eds.). (1994). *Moral development in the professions: Psychology and applied ethics*. Hillsdale, NJ: Lawrence Erlbaum Associates, Publishers.

Rochon, S. (1993). Assessment in rehabilitation. Course material Clinical Behavioral Sciences: Fundamentals of Rehabilitation Course, Department of Psychiatry, McMaster University, Hamilton, Ontario.

Rochon, S. (1994). *Theory from practice: A reflective curriculum for occupational therapists*. Unpublished Master's thesis. Hamilton, ON: McMaster University.

Rochon, S., & Worth, B. (1995). Working together to meet the challenges of change: A transitions workshop for middle managers. Unpublished.

Spelman, E. V. (1977). On treating persons as persons. *Ethics, 88,* 150-161.

Spencer, L.J. [for The Institute of Cultural Affairs] (1989). *Winning through participation: Meeting the challenge of corporate change with the technology of participation: The group facilitation methods of the Institute of Cultural Affairs*. Dubuque, IA: Kendall/Hunt Publishing Co.

Sugarman, L. (1986). *Life span development: Concepts, theories and interactions*. New York: Methuen & Co. Ltd.

Waxler-Morrison, N., Anderson, J., & Richardson, E. (1990). *Cross-cultural caring: A handbook for health professionals in Western Canada*. Vancouver, BC: University of British Columbia Press.

Weiner, B. (1992). *Human motivation: metaphors, theories and research*. Newbury Park, CA: Sage Publications.

Yerxa, E. J. (1983). Audacious values: The energy source for occupation therapy. In G. Kielhofner (Ed.). *Health through occupation: Theory and practice in occupational therapy*. Philadelphia: F. A. Davis Co, pp. 149-162.

Yerxa, E. J. (1992). Some implications of occupational therapy's history for its epistemology, values and relation to medicine. *American Journal of Occupational Therapy, 46*(1), 79-83.

INDEX